"A raw and compelling i[illegible]us psychiatric care that left me reeling—and utterly in[illegible] of the strength of the human spirit. A life-affirming book full of hope, courage and adventure."

Jon Stock
Author of 'The Sleep Room'

"A brave, eloquent and unflinchingly honest memoir of abuse, trauma, incarceration and acute mental distress, which turns on a hinge onto a world of healing, freedom and the transformative power of love."

Nicci Gerrard
Novelist and author of 'What Dementia Teaches Us About Love'

"This is a powerful book. It demonstrates Clare's strength, determination and power to her own truth to have been able to overcome her horrific experiences of her past to become the accomplished woman she is. A must read for anyone who finds themselves in a difficult place facing their own struggles, and anyone who wants to read an uplifting book about overcoming life's challenges and struggles to find a better place in the world."

Emma Jones
Partner in human rights department

"I came to know Clare Allcard very well while researching my biography of her foster son, Thomas Tangvald, and during that time she shared with me, in thumbnail form, the story of her early life. I was amazed then at how well she had coped with the trauma of those years and how open she was about it. Now, having read this book, which describes her ordeal in gripping, dramatic detail, I am utterly blown away. To state it baldly: Clare Allcard is one of the most remarkable people I have ever met, and here—at last—is the full tale of how she became that person. The story, I can assure you, is every bit as remarkable as she is."

Charles J. Doane
Cruising Editor at SAIL Magazine and author of 'The Boy Who Fell to Shore: The Extraordinary Life and Mysterious Disappearance of Thomas Thor Tangvald'

"Clare's story is beautifully told. I like her writing style. At times I was annoyed with some of the attitudes portrayed and at others I was near to tears. The different environments which Clare found herself in were familiar. I could give an in-depth assessment but that's not my task here. Overall she portrays well the lot of the revolving door type of patient—a nasty cliche—for those with multiple admissions to the psychiatric service. I'm so glad to hear that she has her life together now.

From my professional point of view I would like to add that, whilst in the midst of serious mental illness the inherent and ongoing changes clinically, professionally and politically are outwith the sufferers concern. This is not to blame anyone, especially not the sufferer, but the reality is that these changes were ongoing from the '60s onwards. They were particularly active at St Francis Hospital."

Joe Hughes
Former psychiatric nurse at St Francis Hospital and author of 'My Asylum'

From the Devil to the Deep Blue Sea

to Emma,

with thanks for all

the work you do

towards more

effective & compassionate

care

& best wishes

Lidia

To my beloved Edward
who saved my life
and
to our daughter, Kate,
who brought us so much joy.
Rest in Peace.

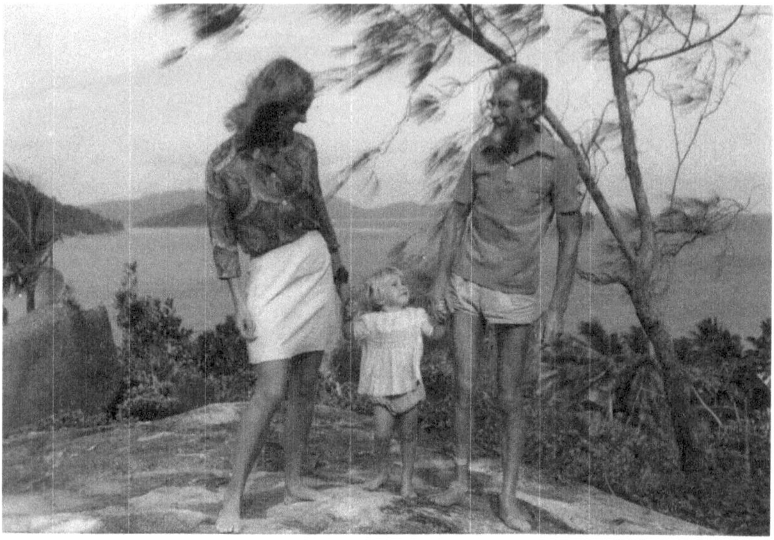

Clare, Kate and Edward in the Seychelles.

From the Devil to the Deep Blue Sea

Clare Allcard

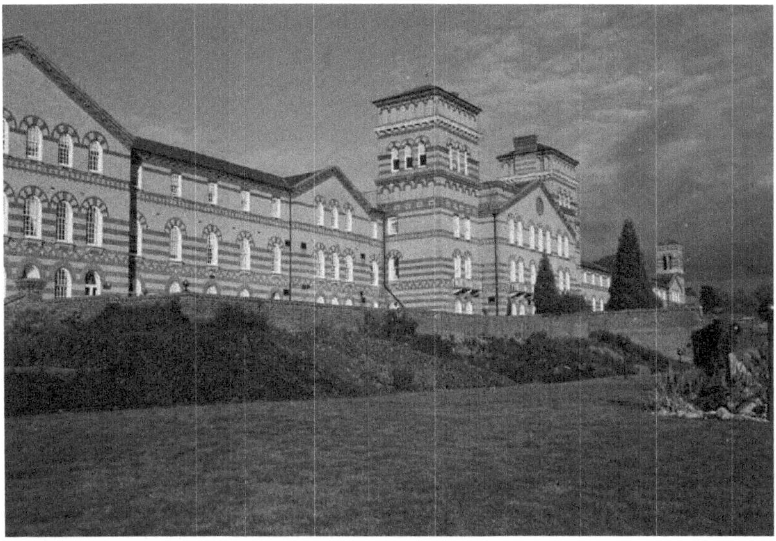

St Francis Hospital.

GOLDEN DUCK

First edition published 2025 by Golden Duck (UK) Ltd
Sokens, Green Street, Pleshey, nr Chelmsford, Essex, CM3 1HT
golden-duck.co.uk

A CIP catalogue record for this book
is available from the British Library

ISBN 978-1-899262-69-4

Printed and bound in the UK by Biddles Books Ltd
biddles.co.uk

Contents

Series Editor's Introduction

"BY THE TIME I was 21," writes Clare Allcard, "I'd already failed to be an actress or a nurse and was instead fully occupied in being a wreck." In 1968, confined in the women's ward in an old-fashioned county asylum,[i] she came across a *Sunday Express* article about a man sailing the world alone, daring to live out his dreams. Clare wrote him a fan letter. "I told the man that I too could think of nothing more fabulous than to sail away into the pale blue yonder, but that there was this one slight snag: I happened to be locked up in a loony bin."

Lone circumnavigator Edward Allcard sent an encouraging reply, telling her to hurry up and get well. He suggested that she might find an ocean voyage monotonous, "but when I am nearer an interesting cruising ground, I would consider it an honour to take you for a trip." Many years later, when Clare came to write her autobiography *A Gypsy Life* (1992) she focused on the travels undertaken together from 1974, the year Edward completed his solo circumnavigation and they bought the Baltic ketch *Johanne Regina* as a home for themselves and their young daughter, Katy. She said nothing more about the events that had led her to be compulsorily detained under Section 25 of the Mental Health Act 1959.

The truth about Clare's experience before she wrote that letter to Edward was eventually made public by her friend, Charles Doane, when he was writing about her foster son, the troubled teenager Thomas Tangvald (*The Boy Who Fell to Shore* 2022). The prolonged silence was not intentional. Clare had written this book, her account of her experience in the 1960s English mental health system, immediately after completing her two commissioned sailing books in the 1990s. The Judge's comment in the 1986 Ealing Vicarage Rape Case, "Her trauma was not too great," had infuriated her and given the courage to tell her own story of rape and trauma. "I believe the more these taboos are spoken about openly, the sooner the shame will shift from the victim to the perpetrator," she wrote later.

But despite the sales success of *A Gypsy Life* and her previous book *The Intricate Art of Living Afloat*, no one was willing to publish this book, then tentatively entitled *A Story of Hope*. It was put aside—to the particular disappointment of Clare's step-daughter, artist Dona Mackereth, who had supported her when she was writing it, together with Clare's husband (Dona's father) Edward and their daughter Kate.

Twenty years later, when I was researching *Stars to Steer By*, Charles Doane introduced me to Clare. I was already an admirer of *A Gypsy Life* and assumed that her reticence in the earlier book was deliberate, that she didn't want to tell the full truth. I was astounded when she sent me the complete typescript of *A Story of Hope*. I read it in a sitting, gripped by the narrative itself and Clare's honesty and intelligence relating it. With each re-reading I find more to admire—the descriptions of the hospitals in which she was an involuntary patient, the pen portraits of her fellow patients and, above all, her ability to describe the feeling of inner evil that had persuaded her it was her duty to kill herself.

Clare carries the reader with her as the factors leading to her first suicide attempt accumulate. There is the rape itself and the perverse success with which she buries the memory so deep that she consciously forgets it. There are also the unsupported encounters with death in the early years of her nurse's training, the arrogant sexist mockery of the medical students, the fear of schizophrenia and, perhaps most insidiously of all, the experience of chronic pain and its belittlement by medical professionals. No one can truly feel another's pain but the least we should offer is acceptance and respect—and, ideally, effective analgesics.

From the Devil to the Deep Blue Sea (thank you Dona Mackereth for the title) takes us back to the mental health world of the mid-1960s. The rules of consent were different then, relatively recently defined by the 1959 Mental Health Act. Clare, aged 19, had no rights. Only her parents could give consent for treatment. Her mother's letter, quoted at the end of this narrative, shows how bewildered they had felt in the hands of the psychiatrists. From a medical perspective Clare was being treated in the wake of the earlier c20th 'heroic' period—where, as Jon Stock explains in *The Sleep Room* (The Bridge Street Press 2025) it was the doctor who thought he (not usually she) was the hero, with his (not usually her) readiness to utilise dramatic, often physical interventions—ECT, deep narcosis, lobotomy—primarily on female patients. Physical restraints were gone (usually) but by the mid-1960s psychopharmacy (usually Largactil) was another ready weapon in the psychiatric armoury. For this edition, a section has been added after the conclusion of the original manuscript, *A Story of Hope*, using other, more recent, writing by Clare to bring the narrative up to the present day, and allow her to reflect on her experience as she approaches her 80th birthday.

One can read Clare's story as history, an eloquent and potentially important testimony from a patient, a voice professionals need to hear—now as then. Most, but not all, of the hospitals in which she was treated no longer exist, others have lost their records. Some institutions may wish to deny their own history or their involvement in now-discredited or damaging treatments. But when history is not attended to, its harms may be repeated. Looking at the various hospitals/units/asylums in which Clare was treated, so many of them had been founded with the most humane and enlightened intentions, only to be reduced by financial stringency, overcrowding and, perhaps, compassion fatigue. Yet they are part of our history and should not be casually dismissed. We have therefore included additional information in the notes and bibliography. Royal College of Psychiatrists honorary archivist Claire Hilton writes: "I think that the blanketing of former mental hospitals as wholly bad (which they weren't) is unhelpful for policy makers, doctors and managers today as it instils a sense of complacency that 'we are better than them', which is ultimately harmful to patients today."[ii] Linda Gask's recent study *Out of Her Mind* (Cambridge University Press 2024) includes examples of inhumane treatment, inflicted today, that would not seem out of place in Barbara Robb's famous exposé *Sans Everything* (1967). Patients' and relatives' voices are currently (summer 2025) being heard in the Lampard Inquiry and the tales that they have to tell are not comfortable to hear.

The physical existence of the huge 19th- and 20th-century county asylums, such as St Francis, Haywards Heath, near Clare's childhood home, might emotionally overshadow their localities. In *Bullet* (Granta 2024), Tom Lee quotes Diana Gittins' description of the old asylums as "little known or understood, though much feared, where each and every individual might, if they were not careful, or if luck failed them, end up".[iii] Our corresponding 21st century fear may be ending up homeless, sleeping on the street. 'Care in the community' reforms have not yet been an unqualified improvement.

All the names of Clare's fellow patients have been changed but not all names of staff. Clare deeply resented the power of the medical establishment, yet she is never rude about the nurses who care for her. She had experience as a psychiatric nurse herself and is quick to recognise acts of kindness, such as the male nurse (regrettably unnamed) who picked the thorns out of her bare feet after she had tried to run away. It has been a piece of great good fortune to be able to speak to psychiatric nurse, Joe Hughes, author of *My Asylum* (Bothán Productions 2015) and his wife Maura, also a nurse. Joe began working at the Villa and St Francis main building from 1967, around the time Clare was a patient there, and Maura arrived in 1968.

Clare was fundamentally frightened of her psychiatrists—even when she could see that they were trying to help—and could feel both defensive and hostile towards them. Her resistance was not only to the treatments that were practised on her but to the questioning which felt threateningly intrusive and one-sided. She became hyper-aware of the 'sanity table' which separated the professional in (almost always) his position of power, from her, the patient, who was to be interrogated and helped to change.

In resisting them she felt she was in a battle for her mind.

Health professionals today often feel the need to insist that they don't come to work to do a bad job. To quote Claire Hilton again, the tendency to look back and indulge in blanket criticism of past practice may be unfair. "In the process many good people who tried their utmost to help people have been overlooked and, I think, wronged in the process." She suggests that the retention of professionals' real names is "part of righting a harmful stereotype". That has usually been our practice here and, where possible, we have added a little extra information in the endnotes. However, in two cases where Clare makes specific accusations, which at this distance cannot be substantiated, we have changed the person's name.

Clare's time in the mental health system was sixty years ago. She was 19 then. From the day she left England aged 22, to this day living in Andorra, she has led a life of unusual variety and adventure. When I asked her for a single special memory of her sailing years, she sent this:

And I do have one glorious memory on Johanne. *She was 98ft long if you count the bowsprit. All sails set. Me totally alone at the helm. Sun setting and a line squall on the horizon, heading towards us and, for the first time, I decided to 'do it alone' and not call Edward for help. I watched the rain pounding on the sea, the white crests whipped up by the wind advancing towards me as I gently eased the bow to port to catch the full force of the wind on the jibs and main. And then the amazing exhilaration when the wind struck and 99 tonnes of ancient oak leaped forward across the ocean and we charged towards the setting sun. And I was in control...*

What a contrast to her time in the asylums where "you have no autonomy, no control at all". Although *Between the Devil and the Deep Blue Sea* is in many ways not a regular Golden Duck title, it may reflect the experience of many others who have suffered from PTSD or other mental illness and who find deep healing at sea. Many years later, Clare responded strongly to Ed Gorman's *Death of a Translator* (Arcadia 2017), in which the former foreign correspondent reflects on the solace he found working on his boat, and sailing.[iv]

This book is also a love story—so thank you, Dona Mackereth, for focussing in your Foreword on the lifelong happiness which your father and Clare gave one another.

We are grateful to Charles Doane, Emma Jones, Emma Wolverson, Claire Hilton, Jon Stock, Joe and Maura Hughes for their knowledge and advice; to Dona Mackereth for the front cover design, Pere Alemany from Amics del Quetx Ciutat de Badalona for recent photographs of *Johanne Regina* (and for the care they take of her as their sail training ship today) and to Joe Hughes for photographs of buildings which Clare rarely saw from the outside.

Above all I would like to express my personal admiration for Clare. Thirty years on from the time this book was written, she now has some short-term memory problems to contend with but her determination to tell and understand the truth of what happened to her between 1965–1968 remains undimmed, as does her fluency with her pen. She wrote this book both for herself and for others who may have experienced powerlessness, trauma, disbelief and cycles of undeserved self-loathing. I only wish that all her fellow patients in those 1960s institutions could have achieved such a happy ending.

Julia Jones
Peter Duck, 2025

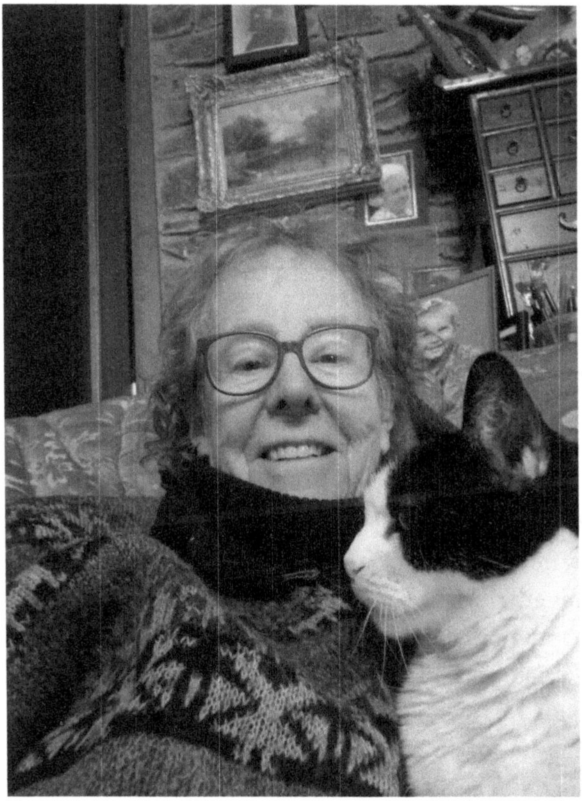

Clare and Meri.

Foreword

I WAS ASKED TO give a speech at my dad's 100th birthday party. I asked my sister, Kate for her reminiscences of our father and they were about how much she had loved learning from him. When Clare answered the same question her response was very brief. "He saved my life". Remember those words when you come to the end of this book.

I was living in Singapore in a basher hut with a girlfriend, on the edge of the jungle, when a letter arrived from my Dad. You can tell it was quite a few years ago, no email. He mentioned that he would be driving through Singapore en route to New Zealand, with a fellow traveller called Clare. Could we meet up? Absolutely. They came to collect me in the Land Rover and we drove to a hotel for a meal. On the way Clare was navigating through the very frustrating Singapore roads, and suddenly shouted to Edward "no darling you need to turn left". That told me everything! And I was happy for them.

Clare was two years younger than me, but it never occurred to me that it was a bit odd for there to be such a large age gap between Edward and Clare. (He and my mother had been separated for several years.) The following evening they came for supper with me and several friends, and we had a wonderful evening.

They departed from Singapore by ship to New Zealand and Edward continued to write to me over the following years. He was such a great letter writer, and later email correspondent. Apart from my earlier years when Edward was around, he and I had communicated by letter. He was an intermittent presence in my life, but certainly a very significant one.

We next met up about eight years later! They had sailed their boat, *Johanne Regina*, back to the UK, from the Seychelles, and were berthed in Lymington Marina. My partner and I went to visit them and asked the harbour master for directions, he suggested we just look for the largest boat in the marina! This was my first introduction to *Johanne*, and my second meeting with Clare.

Edward was patient, calm, thoughtful, and compassionate. These qualities brought them together at a time when Clare was very vulnerable. How extraordinary it is that they met, in such odd circumstances, and that there was a miraculous happy ending. How lucky we both were, me to have a very special father, and Clare to find the love of her life.

Dona Mackereth

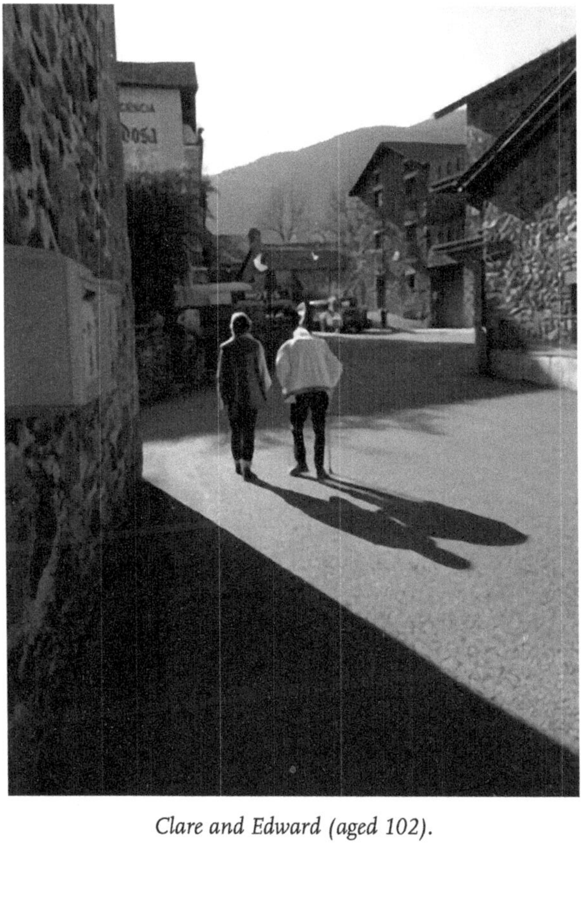

Clare and Edward (aged 102).

PART ONE

FROM THE DEVIL

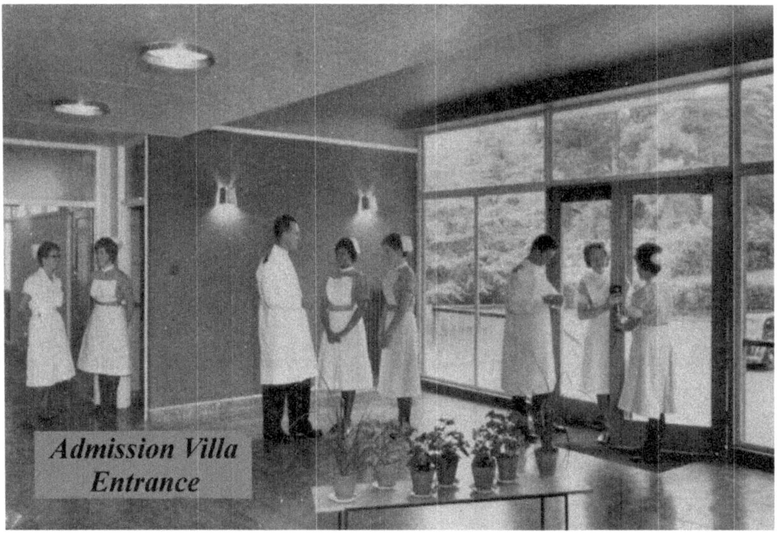

The Villa. [Credit: Joe Hughes]

1

The Final Straw

The year was 1965. The Stones could get no satisfaction. Mary Quant introduced the miniskirt. The Post Office Tower opened. London rocked. And I was a cheery, 19-year-old extrovert in my second year, training to be a nurse at London's Middlesex Hospital.

Then, one night, I went to the cinema alone. I was a student nurse on a psychiatric secondment[v] and I liked doing things alone. I was already halfway back to the nurses' hostel when I heard footsteps approaching from behind.

"Hey! Stop! Wait a minute!" A man's voice echoed up the empty street.

Lamplight glistened on the wet pavement. A hint of fog hung in the air and prickled around my wavy hair. I quickened my pace, striding over the damp leaves, head high, wishing now that I wasn't quite so completely alone.

"Oh come on. Can't yer stop! I want to talk to yer."

His breathing sounded laboured, as if he was hurrying to catch up. The Woodside Psychiatric unit's nurses' hostel lay just around the corner. Maybe I should make a dash for it. Then I slowed. Wasn't this what my life was supposed to be about: listening to people? Hadn't I said to my friend that very morning, "I reckon half our so called 'psychiatric' patients aren't sick at all; just desperately lonely"? Yet here I was, a few hours later, fleeing to safety while the person behind me could be suicidal.

The next time he called, "Stop!" I stopped, then turned to face downhill towards him. I watched as he approached: a big man in his mid-thirties with broad shoulders, dark hair and large hands. Hands had always fascinated me. I loved my father's hands: expressive, soft and cushiony.

"I was sitting next t'yer in the cinema," he panted. "Do yer want to come out for a drink?"

I peered into his shadowed eyes, trying to probe past them into his mind. Was he sick? Lonely? Desperate?

"I'm awfully sorry but I've got to get back. I'm late already." I made a show of looking at my watch, not wanting to hurt his feelings. "And you know, I don't think we sat next to each other in the cinema."

"Oh, come on! Please! Just a quick one."

I hesitated. I couldn't remember him in the cinema. But surely that was irrelevant. The question was, how can you say in the morning that half the world's mental illness is due to loneliness and then, come nightfall, deny the first cry for help? Of course, the religious teachers at my last school had always warned us against speaking to strange men—let alone going for a drink with one! But hadn't they also taught compassion? Hadn't they repeated Saint Paul's words, "Clothe yourselves with compassion, kindness, humility, gentleness and patience?" Wasn't that even more important?

"Okay. If you really want." My voice wavered, reluctant, regretting my decision even as I made it.

The man led the way to a beat-up van. "In yer get. We'll try a new place I've heard of." He wrenched the door open with difficulty and helped me up into the cab.

As we drove, I squinted apprehensively through the thickening fog but was soon totally lost. Leaning back on the hard, plastic-covered seat, I tried to look nonchalant, mature. Absently I hugged my right arm where chronic pain had begun one of its frequent bouts, burrowing deep into the bone. The more the man talked the more foolish I felt. He was nothing like our normally listless, medicated, male patients. Indeed, his raw self-confidence intimidated me. Concentrating hard to decipher his words above the engine, I was shocked when, suddenly, the phantom, fog-wrapped streetlights disappeared entirely.

"Hey! Where are we going?" I turned to face him, scared. "Take me back! They'll lock me out if I'm not back by midnight!"

"Don't worry, Cinderella, this 'ere's a short cut. You'll get back okay."

"But where are we?"

The man chuckled; then rammed the wheel hard over. The van

bounded up the kerb. I flew forward, grabbed the dashboard. We jolted across rough ground and came to a halt beside a high hedge; a dark, menacing hedge. He switched off the engine.

I seized my door handle and jerked it hard. It wouldn't budge! I had to escape! Desperately, I hit the door with my fists even as I felt the man lean towards me in the dark. Heard him laugh softly, "Hampstead Heath mi' lovely!"

Then he put his hands around my throat and gently squeezed. I believed I was going to die. Facing death. He was going to kill me right there.

"Now get in the back!" he whispered in my ear. In the back? I looked. There, in the back, rolled to one side, was a long beige blanket. My petrified mind seized on it, stared at it, hypnotised. He was going to wrap my dead body in it, I knew he was! Then hide it and me under the hedge!

And then he raped me.

Next morning, I almost told my best friend in the hostel what had happened. But found I couldn't. I was too ashamed. Ashamed of my naive stupidity. Instead, I stuffed the whole memory deep inside me and slammed the manhole cover shut. Only a dark feeling of fear and maybe evil gave witness to the fact that something seismic had happened in my life.

Buried traumas can lead to madness. Now I believe that if I'd had the courage to share that night with one other person, anyone, my later story could possibly have been quite different.[vi]

* * *

"Right, I think that's all." Sister Forbes closed the ward's card file and, morning report over, got up from her desk. "Oh no! One more thing. They need volunteers down in the lab. Some sort of adrenaline research. If any of you want to take part let me know and you can go off early."

My ears pricked up. I'd always been intensely curious. "I'll go, Sister," I said, my voice touched with excitement. "Could be interesting."

"Fine." Sister smiled approvingly. "Eleven o'clock? You know where it is, Nurse Thompson?" I nodded, setting my absurd, 19th century, nurses' starched headgear bouncing.

The labs, like the rest of the psychiatric unit, showed signs of exhaustion: chipped brown linoleum stretched below grubby, mushroom-coloured walls.

I hesitated at the door of a side room, scanning the gloom. The place looked like a small torture chamber: a wooden, straight-backed armchair for the victim, linked up to an alarming array of wires. Hell! Any year now I'd learn not to leap feet first into situations just because they sounded 'interesting'.

"Hi! Come on in. What's your name?"

"Rosemary Clare Thompson—but everyone calls me Clare."

"Clare it is then. I'm Mark. Has anyone told you what we're doing?" His hair was dark, thick and curly.

"Only that it's something to do with adrenaline."

"Right. Well, the idea is to see whether psychiatric patients have a greater sense of fear, or maybe imagination, than the normal population. You're supposed to represent the latter." When he laughed the corners of his eyes crinkled into tiny crows' feet. "What we do is couple you up to these wires: this here measures respiration, this one skin tension, this sweat and this one pulse. Once you're wired up, I want you to think of something that you're a bit frightened of... Got any suggestions?"

My mind went completely blank.

"What about the dentist?"

"Well, I suppose so. Yes, okay." I couldn't really see that it mattered.

"Right. Now. How about some big thing that you're frightened of? Everybody has at least one."

Yes. There was something. I knew there was. I could even feel it, clawing deep inside me. But for the life of me I couldn't remember what. My mind refused to go there.

"What about heights? Afraid of heights at all?"

"Yes. Yes, why not? Not mad on heights."

"Good. So, if you'll sit here, I'll just rig you up." His smile warmed his eyes. Psychiatric nurses are taught to notice these things. "None of this hurts, you know. It's just for measuring reactions."

The conducting gel felt cold on my arms and chest. Using sticky plaster, he strapped on the wires then left the room.

"Can you hear me?" His voice crackled over an intercom into the darkened room.

"Yup."

"Right. Now I want you to relax. Imagine yourself on a lovely beach soaking up the sun."

I stirred uneasily in the hard, upright chair. The ruddy pain was back, gnawing at my arm.

"What's the matter? You're not relaxing."

"Your beach's full of pebbles!" I joked. We laughed and fell silent.

"Okay. That's better. Now I want you to imagine you're in the dentist's waiting room. It's your turn next. The door is opening, the receptionist is..."

I ignored his attempts to alarm me. Instead I thought to myself, *Moderate fear.* Always seeking excitement, it was a trick I'd devised as a child in search of what I later learnt was an adrenaline high. I used to frighten myself deliberately by making hideous faces in the mirror, and then, imagined the face belonged to someone else, peering over my shoulder. Later I'd discarded the mirror altogether and did it all in my head.

The voice over the intercom purred with satisfaction. For my part, I was amused to find I hadn't lost my knack.

"Good! Good! That's great. Now I want you to go back to the beach. Relax. That's right, relax completely. Excellent! Now you're climbing up the stairs of the Post Office Tower. Up! Up! Up! You're getting higher and higher. Now you're right at the top. You're stepping out onto the balcony. You're leaning against the outer safety wall. You're leaning over. You're looking down. The safety barrier is giving way...!'

His voice reached a crescendo, but I wasn't really listening. In my mind I was thinking *Fear! Fear! Fear!* And somewhere my soul screamed back, *Help! Help! Please someone help me!* But the room remained silent.

Now the voice over the intercom sounded alarmed.

"It's okay! You're alright! Hang on, we've got you! It's alright!"

The door flew open, the light flashed on, and a distraught young man rushed in.

"My God! Are you okay?"

I smiled rather sheepishly and blushed.

"Boy, you had me scared for a moment there!" Mark tittered nervously as he disconnected the wires and coiled them up neatly. Clearly he didn't like things to be out of control. Then, as my eyes laughed at him, his enthusiasm returned. "Do you want to see it? See what you did to the graphs?"

Still on edge, I followed him down the corridor to the nerve centre of the laboratory. There, on a draftsman's table, lay a huge sheet of graph paper covered in black lines, most of them rising and falling within certain parameters. All but one. The last one. He jabbed excitedly at it with his finger.

"Look at that! It's incredible! Are you sure you're okay? Look. Here's the nearest thing to your pulse. See? It's about half your rate and that's a patient's. You do realise you've mucked up the whole thing, don't you? Still, it's pretty damned amazing."

"Hey Tom, come and look at this! It's incredible! I was telling her she was falling off the top of the Post Office Tower."

Furtively I checked my pulse. It was still racing too fast to count. And it had absolutely nothing to do with the Post Office Tower.

* * *

The next months of training passed in a whirl of activity: new friends, free tickets to London's top playhouses, shopping at Biba's trendy new boutique where the changing rooms were divided by hessian cloth curtains, weekend train rides back home to my parents to relax after long hours on the wards.

Spring slipped unnoticed into summer. I moved from Woodside back to the main Middlesex Hospital just behind Oxford Street and was now working on Men's Medical. Outside, the city had grown oppressive under its haze of pollution, but inside, the hospital was blessedly cool.

Life was good.

Until, one day, I found myself all alone on an almost empty ward cleared for redecorating. Only three patients remained: all of them too sick to move.

I was sitting beside old Mr Simons. Propped up in bed, unconscious, he caught his breath in feeble gasps through the tracheotomy cut in his throat. He had no relatives, or at least none that visited him. I took his parchment-thin hand and gently massaged it. Over the weeks I'd grown fond of him. Maybe, through the dark, subterranean lake of his unconscious, he could sense the flow of affection I yearned to wrap him in. Maybe he knew someone was there to make sure he didn't face the climax of his life, his death, alone.

I glanced around at the other patients, anxiously checking. With little more than a year's nursing experience, I had been left alone in charge of three near-corpses. Was it a compliment? Did they think I was good at coping with death? Or was it that here I could do no further harm? Some of my friends still hadn't laid out a single body, still hadn't witnessed the 'happy release', the 'great reaper', the 'final sleep'; all those cheating euphemisms I so despised. Yet wherever I went, death seemed to follow. The fear haunted me that somehow it was me; that I was inadvertently killing them off; I was to blame. And always it was the ones I cared about most that died.

Like Peter and Jon, identical seven-year-old twins afflicted with an identical congenital heart defect. The instant Peter died in a room down the corridor, Jon flung himself, frail and sobbing, into my skirts. Without seeing his brother, Jon had known the exact moment at which he'd died. I'd scooped him up in my arms and held him tight, rubbing my lips against his silky blond hair, crooning hushed comforts as my own tears flowed unheeded, adolescent tears of rage at the injustice of life.

Guiltily, my thoughts snapped back to Mr Simons. I shifted his hand in mine and began to talk softly to him. Abruptly, violently, the old man shot forward. His eyes still closed, he gasped. Air rattled in his lungs. A horrifying stream of stinking green slime gushed from the hole in his throat and frothed down his emaciated chest. I snatched up the sucker.

Clumsily, in panic, I thrust its thin hose down his tracheotomy to draw out the phlegm from his lungs, but I was too late. Mr Simons' lifeless body flopped back, his lungs drowned in putrid gunge.

I hesitated a long time before lifting the phone, bracing myself to repeat the student nurses' formula which hospital rules imposed.

"Sister? This is Nurse Thompson on Newark Ward. I think Mr Simons has stopped breathing." Not waiting for a reply, I gently replaced the receiver. Only a doctor knew enough to say that Mr Simons was dead.

* * *

The autumn sky hung low, gently mizzling rain on passers-by. Grey-faced pedestrians glanced in disapproval as I strode past them, my wavy hair uncovered, my psychedelic mac open to reveal a black miniskirt riding high on my thighs. I rebelled against the way everyone was supposed to turn up their coat collars and look miserable; why cower from the rain? Country bred, I liked it. I liked to feel it tingle in my hair and trickle softly down my cheeks.

A couple of days ago, I'd spotted a small advertisement in *The Times* for a public lecture on "Creative Listening" and, curiosity tweaked, took myself off, alone, to investigate. The hall was packed. Dr Rachel Pinney, the lecturer, was a psychotherapist as well as an ardent anti-nuclear activist, later to camp out at Greenham Common.[vii] She saw Creative Listening, or "Listening for Peace", as a solution to the lack of understanding across the nuclear/anti-nuclear divide. That evening those present sat in pairs, facing each other with their opposing views. But only one of us was allowed to speak. The other had to remain silent. This meant one had to concentrate entirely on what the other person had to say. The following week there was going to be a return match with a reversal of roles.

In the odd way that such things happen, at least to me, that night I had ended up in a pub along with Dr Pinney and some of her colleagues. Exhilarated by the discussion, I had accepted the invitation to today's lunch. Indeed, I'd been rather flattered to think that I, a mere student nurse, had captured the lecturer's interest.

Eventually, as I walked, the shops petered out to be superseded by terraced houses. Now I consulted a slip of paper where directions had been written in a large, scraggly hand. I scanned the faces of the old buildings for their numbers, looked up at the front of a tall tenement. What had been an exciting prospect the night before now seemed daunting. I was no longer so sure I wanted to go in, at least not alone. There was something overpowering, something strange about the doctor. Worse, though, would be to be spotted by her as I hesitated outside. So, I climbed the front steps and rang the bell. In a distant recess I heard it clang. Then came the flop slop of slippers on bare wood stairs and the door opened.

A cigarette hung loosely from Dr Pinney's upper lip. Her hair, short cropped, pudding basin-style, had clearly not been touched since she got up that morning. Eyes puckered against smoke, the doctor plucked the cigarette from her mouth and smiled.

"Clare! Come on in."

Despite her eccentricities, Dr Pinney quickly put me at my ease over coffee and sandwiches in the kitchen. Then she led me into the living room. "Come and let me show you my diagnostic equipment. It's outrageously expensive but most effective. I'm trying to develop my own version along the same lines but much cheaper. Why don't you have a go at it?"

A heavy, carved table stood four-square on the worn carpet, its surface hidden deep in papers. Using her forearm, the doctor cleared a swathe then pulled out a chair for me to sit on. Crossing to a mahogany chest of drawers, she collected a wooden box and a square wooden tray.

"Look! Here's the equipment. Six different shaped triangles, each one in a different colour. All you have to do is arrange them in any way you like inside this tray." And she put it down on the table. "Any way you like. It doesn't matter. There is no right or wrong way."

I knew she was lying. There must be a right and wrong way. Unless, of course, all ways were wrong; like the old in-joke: if a patient arrives early for psychotherapy he's suffering from anxiety, if late he's showing his aggression and if on time, then the poor man's clearly obsessive. I began to choose triangles with great care, wondering what hidden portent each one conveyed.

The smell of tobacco warned of the older woman's proximity.

"You know that's most interesting," she said. "Carry on."

I wiped my hands on my skirt then shifted some of the triangles around. I didn't want to be interesting. Even my usual teenage desire to be different had vanished. Right now, I wanted to be totally ordinary.

Unable to stall any longer, I put the last triangle into the tray. Again, she leaned over, closer now.

"As I said, that really is most interesting. Wait and I'll show you."

She crossed once more to the chest of drawers and rummaged amongst the disorder. I tried to focus on the general chaos as proof to myself of her incompetence.

Dr Pinney straightened with a grunt of satisfaction and turned around, a card in her hand. She stopped beside a chair a little distance from me, hesitated and then appeared to decide not to sit down.

She looked at me for a moment then half-turned to stare out of the window. "To be honest with you, Clare," she said, glancing down at her hands, "I'm not quite sure what I should do." She fingered the card absently. "If you were my patient, it would be easy, but you're not." The doctor turned then. "You see, I think you need help. Tell me, have you ever had a nervous breakdown?"

Far away, a monitor in my mind criticised the woman's style. *My dear doctor, that is not the sort of thing you should say to a guest!* But close at hand I heard only the watery rush of fear in my ears, fuelled by acute embarrassment.

"No." Infuriatingly, my voice came out husky. I cleared my throat. "No. Why?" Deeply uncomfortable, I forced myself to return look for look, to let a faintly amused smile touch my lips.

"Clare, I don't usually do this." The doctor again twisted the card between her fingers. "But I probably won't be seeing you again. I must tell you, I think you're on the verge of a nervous breakdown. I also think that you'll probably be schizophrenic within the year."

I felt myself blush furiously. What polite, middle-class formula was one supposed to use in reply to that?

"If you were my patient," she continued, "I would put you top of my list to see a psychoanalyst." She came over. "Look carefully at your pattern."

I looked.

"Now compare it with this." Like a magician, she flourished the selected card.

Approaching it warily, I noted clinically that the card was tatty, its edges fluffed up like some soiled playing card bent with much use. I wondered how many other, nervous, sweaty hands had clasped this grubby denunciation of their sanity. Finally, I dared to look at the bold black capitals centred at the foot of the card:

FIRST STAGES OF SCHIZOPHRENIA

My eyes flew, aghast, to the pattern of triangles above the inscription and then to the tray spread out naked before us. The two were identical, in every possible detail of position, colour and shape. It was devilish rubbish, a freak, like Tarot cards or a Ouija board! Still the printed words came at me, so black and unrelenting, so confident of their credibility: **FIRST STAGES OF SCHIZOPHRENIA.**

"It's nothing to be ashamed of, Clare," Dr Pinney said gently. "If Jesus Christ was alive today they'd treat him for schizophrenia, too. But you must get help, and soon."

"Okay, Dr Pinney." Pushing back my chair, I stood up. I had to get away. "I'll see what I can do. I'm afraid I must go now. I'm on duty soon." I made a show of looking at my watch. Fleetingly, a memory stirred, then was gone. "Thank you so much for the sandwiches. They were delicious."

I left the house determined to forget the doctor and her childish games. Clearly the woman was mad. No psychiatrist in her right mind would say a thing like that. Anyway, the whole system was a load of nonsense.

On the return journey, I became conscious once more of people staring at me. Was it perhaps written on my countenance, what the doctor had said? I hung my head letting my hair fall forward to hide my face.

*   *   *

It seemed no time before Christmas loomed. A rumour travelled like wildfire around the nurses' home. The hospital's new, modernising matron had given permission for us student nurses to take part in the medical students' Christmas show. A date for auditions was posted on the notice board and I was one of the first to sign up. Not only because I loved acting but also because I'd heard that one of the junior doctors, Ben, was the director. I quite fancied him.

The audition's judges, four medical students, sat in the front row of the stalls while we hopefuls milled around on stage. First, we had to mime a scene. I was instructed to present a person who goes into an unfamiliar, pitch-dark room, finds the light switch, and, on spinning round, discovers a dead body.

After my Marcel Marceau-inspired miming performance, Ben asked, "Can you scream?"

"Yes, of course, but it's supposed to be a mime. You don't scream in mime."

"Ah, but I want to hear if you can scream."

Suddenly, weirdly my belly clenched. Why? What fear was this, clinging around a scream?

"You really want me to?" I called out, a slight challenge in my voice.

"Yes!"

"As loud as I can?"

"Yes!"

I'd show them! I summoned every last ounce of energy. Opened my mouth. And SCREAMED. The result was instantaneous and most gratifying: a great round of applause and lots of laughter. I'd done it! I'd screamed! Though why I felt so liberated I couldn't work out.

And so on to the next bit. All of us young women applying for parts had been told by the judges, all young men, to bring along bikinis.

When I was 12, I'd had an excruciating pain in my right side. A surgeon had carved me almost in half, eventually discovering a benign tumour blocking the tube from my kidney to my bladder. He left me with a livid purple scar that ran, half an inch wide, across my body starting just below my ribs. I'd never owned a bikini as I was too mortified by the scar, but I did have a two-piece, tropical beach outfit, a minimalist pair of shorts and matching top. Now, glancing around, I saw I was the only one looking frumpy and old fashioned. Still, at least my legs were svelte enough.

Reluctantly, I lined up with the others as we walked across the stage one by one to be ogled. Humiliating, but not one of us rebelled. Inside I seethed but if I wanted to be in the show then that's what I had to do. Follow the crowd.

Still in our bikinis, we were cross-examined about motivation.

Eventually, Ben turned to me. "So why do you want to be in the show?"

"Because I love acting!"

"That's no good," Ben told me, laughing. "You're supposed to say, 'Because I want to sleep with Roy there.'" And he pointed.

I followed Ben's outstretched arm and saw a young man with dark hair, a bull neck and large hands. He was leering at me. Something inside me sickened. I turned back, repulsed.

"But I don't!" I declared forcefully. I knew, instantly, that I'd said it too loudly and with far too much conviction. The crowd fell into shocked silence while I felt my cheeks yet again flush furiously. Roy was one of the show's leading lights and clearly considered himself God's gift to women. Too late I realised I should have modulated my voice, tried to hide my disgust, not spoken so loudly. Basically not spoken at all. I had publicly humiliated him.

I did get a part in the show—but Roy was out for revenge.

It was one of the other nurses who warned me that he was offering a reward for anyone screwing me before the show ended. Several students invited me out to pubs, presumably hoping to seduce me. Even Ben cornered me one night in a small room backstage, wrapped his arms tight around and forced his tongue into my mouth in a long, wet kiss. My eyes stretched wide with shock as I stared at him, haunted. Ben let me go and left, muttering "Sorry."

And these were to be our future doctors!

The harassment continued throughout the weeks of rehearsals. I said nothing, told no one, but I was damned if I was going to be bullied into leaving. I wouldn't give the jerk that satisfaction.

The script was witty, the show full of songs. Indeed, it was said to be that year's best medical student show in town as it took an irreverent poke at the hospital's top doctors and professors, referring to the newly invented contraceptive pill as the 'sweet with the non-fattening centre'.

Simon was a quiet, highly intelligent, final-year student blessed with a striking baritone voice. As the cast's end-of-show party drew near, he invited me to be his date for the evening. Frankly, I couldn't believe my luck. Only later did I discover that he'd invited me partly out of chivalry and partly in order to spike Roy's chances to score.

A fund-raising album was sold to cover the show's costs. Roy's closing attack came on the back cover where a passport shot of each cast member appeared with a short, affectionate comment beside it. However, next to mine, it said, "Mensa Member. Finds everything *so* boring!" The scorn was patent—and it was patently untrue. It was true that after leaving school at 17, I'd worked as a mother's help on a farm whilst studying for a place at drama school. Seriously bored, I'd seen an advertisement in a newspaper for Mensa, the international, high IQ club. I took the test, did well and was accepted, but I quickly learnt that it was best that you never told anyone you belong to Mensa. It raises instant resentment. As far as I could remember, since coming to London, I'd only ever mentioned it once and that was to George—a friend of Ben's.

Roy had won. Acting euphoria over, the spite and humiliation behind that record cover plunged me into misery.

* * *

Two a.m. and I was still awake. The nights were always the worst. I had tried all the usual remedies: I'd taken painkillers but they hadn't helped, I'd plunged my arm into searing hot water then freezing cold. I'd hugged it and pounded it and dug my nails into it and contorted it. Like a wild animal caught in a trap, I'd tried everything to change the grinding monotony of the pain, a pain that had started when I was 13, one year after the surgery that had left the ugly scar. Pacing back and forth I knew I would eventually fall asleep from sheer exhaustion, as I had done for the past five years; only to be woken again a few hours later by more pain and the prospect of a heavy day's work ahead.

Finally, six weeks ago, a doctor had agreed to perform an exploratory operation. I had been brim-full of hope. To his surprise, though not mine, he had found a congenital defect in the nerve that led to my right arm, and which had grown wrapped around my first rib. Each and every movement of my arm aggravated it. The man had excised the rib—but the pain had actually grown worse. For a while the operation's failure had pitched me into grey-hazed desolation. Gradually I'd fought back, resurfaced. I had decided that, if there was another operation, next time it would be different. Next time I wouldn't hope at all.

Outside, a clock chimed. Another couple of hours and I would be back in hospital for further investigations though it wasn't clear how they would help. Nerves don't show up on x-rays.

Later that day, they wheeled me back from the radiology department on a trolley. By the time my eminent neurosurgeon walked onto the ward I was deep into a book. Feigning nonchalance, I went on reading until he reached the end of my bed. There he picked up my latest results and said to the accompanying ward sister, "These showed no further abnormalities. There's nothing more that can be done. I've written her up for Neulactil for the pain. See she takes it." And without a glance in my direction, he walked away.

Oh, dear God, I had hoped! Of course I had! And now he was telling me I could expect another sixty years of this bloody pain, of sleepless nights and exhausted days. Would they let a dog go through that? Of course not. The owners would be had up by the cruelty people.

For more than an hour I lay quite still as damp tentacles of hopelessness wrapped themselves around my mind. How was I going to carry on? More to the point, why should I? And what was this Neulactil anyway? I'd never heard of it. They'd never used it on any ward I'd worked on. Climbing slowly out of bed, I headed down the corridor to the nurses' station. They'd have a copy of Mimms, the pharmaceutical dictionary. I'd soon know what Neulactil was for. Picking it up I quickly thumbed through the pharmacopoeia. N... Ne... Neulactil!

'Useful in the treatment of acute and chronic schizophrenia...'

* * *

It is said that suicide is most often triggered by the final straw in an accumulation of apparently insoluble situations. Slowly those apparently insoluble situations had accumulated: the humiliation of not being believed by the doctors, the sexual harassment around Roy's victory, the condemnation to lifelong pain, fear of schizophrenia and always that dark, persistent, unidentified terror and revulsion buried deep inside me. But terror of what? That I could not remember.

Around each situation hung an aura of shame. Maybe it was at Tildonk, a Catholic Ursuline convent school in Belgium, that the sense of shame had started, inculcated daily into a group of eleven-year old girls on our knees in chapel. At 6a.m. each morning, we beat our chests declaring, *"Mea culpa! Mea Culpa! Mea maxima culpa!"* "My fault! My Fault! My most grievous fault!"

I was an 'Army brat' and education for itinerant Army kids is always a problem. First my parents tried taking me on every posting and sending me to local schools. But that meant I ended up being educated in nine different places, in two different languages and three different systems. Nevertheless, it taught me how to make friends in double quick time. The alternative was boarding school, offering a stable, continuous education and long-lasting friendships. Some hated it. To me, boarding offered the best of both worlds. I spent all term with my friends and then, by the end of term, I looked forward to returning home to my family for the holidays. Many of the girls at the convent were miserable, but I wasn't. Indeed, when I first went there, aged 10, I was deeply impressed. The place was conducted in full-immersion French and this included the prayers. I remember after a couple of weeks I was beginning to understand a little of the Catholic prayer known in English as The Hail Mary. In French it went "Santa Marie, Mère de Dieu" but to my ears it sounded like Santa Marie Major Jew. I was thrilled! Here was a religion that actually acknowledged that Jesus was Jewish!

Nine years later, beyond the inexplicable shame, it was the Neulactil, pointing to the imminent threat of schizophrenia, that proved to be the final straw. How ghastly for my parents if their bright and cheery and oh-so-stable daughter went mad.

* * *

It took me another month to make the final decision to kill myself. Then I sat in my bedroom in the nurses' home and wrote a letter to my dear, sweet brother, Dave. Three years older than me, he had always been my wise and gentle mentor.

Family letters had featured prominently throughout my life, from my boarding school days in Belgium when, on Thursdays, we daughters of officers of the British Army of the Rhine wrote draft letters home. These were corrected and edited by one of the English-speaking nuns and then, on Saturday mornings, we copied out the results—all complaints redacted—in our fairest hand. They were then posted off to our parents. I would then wait eagerly for my mother's reply. This weekly ritual instilled in me a lifelong habit of letter, and today, email writing.

And it seemed only right that Dave should know and, if possible, understand, what I planned to do—and why. I began in the early hours of February 5th 1966:

Dearest Dave,

I've finally made the decision. I'm going to put myself down.

I've collected a month's repeat prescription of that blessed man's tablets—it seemed fitting. This time they really will "help the pain".

Shame, constant pain, the threat of schizophrenia, tell me what sort of future is that?

Phew! It's not as easy as you think, swallowing quantities of pills. But I've got them down and now I'm just waiting, with my incubus, for sleep. I don't feel at all frightened. I don't feel anything really. Why should I? Isn't fear of death really fear of unbearable pain in the dying, of not knowing when it will come? And maybe simply fear of the unknown. Should we fear hell fire and damnation? I don't think so. Hell is here on earth. That other hell, of flame and brimstone, was invented by a medieval Church in order to maintain control over a large, illiterate peasantry. No. This way I'm cheating death of its uncertainty and doing everyone a service into the bargain. All those patients I cared for, they will no longer die in rivers of green slime as I stroke their hands—delicate, bird-like hands, Davey, criss-crossed with blue-wormed veins.

For months now I've sensed something evil in me. Something rotten, ready to burst out. Some terrible shame that dear Death will bury with it.

Should I write a separate note to say I want to be cremated? No, you'll tell them won't you? Silly really. I know I'll be dead, but I still don't like the thought of fat maggots humping in and out of my flesh. Ashes scattered to the four winds that's for me.

I love you and Mum, Dad and John above everything, David, remember that. I'm doing this for all of us. And please, be glad that I can sleep in peace at last.

I'm beginning to feel wonderfully warm and drowsy and my eyesight seems to be going. Do you realise, for the first time in years, I'm actually going to fall asleep pain-free! The bastard was quite right, Dave. His pills do stop the pain. His only mistake was the dose...

Your loving sister—always,

Clare

2

Imprisoned

THE IMPATIENT CLANG of sterile stainless steel. Tubes thrust roughly down the throat. Water. Pumps. For a fleeting moment the duty doctor's resentment bruised my consciousness. Then grey oblivion.

Dead? Floating up; up and away? But my spirit could not escape entirely. Like an abandoned child's balloon, it rested in a high corner of the room, disembodied, gazing down on the still life below. That body, lying so stiff under the white sheets, was it really mine? Was that me with the fair hair spread around a white face laid deeply into a white pillow?

Neuroscientists are divided on the cause of out-of-body experiences. Maybe there are various causes depending on the individual, for out-of-body experiences are not that rare.

"Hello, Clare. Can you hear me?" A nurse leant over the body, my body, and shook it tentatively. "How do you feel now?" She moved a strand of hair away from my face—and broke the spell. I could no longer stay apart. My spirit reunited with its body.

Light filtered behind my eyelids and pierced the comfortable darkness of my hiding. I opened my eyes a fraction, putting out tiny feelers into the world.

I wasn't dead.

God! How pathetic can you get? You can't even kill yourself properly! Slowly my brain rallied to my defence, forced me to lie still for fear the nurse might pry into my misery.

Nurse Bowden, a psychiatric nurse in her mid-twenties, stood up, casting a shadow across my closed eyes. Involuntarily, I held my breath, waiting for the first assault upon my sanctuary.

"Clare! Time to wake up!"

Don't touch me! Please! I don't want to wake up. But careful now, they mustn't know or they will keep me here and then I really shall go mad.

I opened my eyes, struggled to focus on the woman standing over me, smiling her well-trained smile. Then I turned my head away, felt my throat raw from their tubes.

"I'm awake," I whispered.

"Good! How are you feeling?"

I didn't answer. All I wanted was for her to go away. To leave me alone.

She paused, then said, "Well then, I'll just tell Sister Will. After that I'll be back with something for you to eat."

My stomach roiled. The mere thought of food made me want to vomit but I would try. I determined to try anything in order to win my release, before they could start delving into the malevolent darkness inside me.

As she left, I put my hand out and groped over the top of the bedside locker, searching for my glasses. Severely short-sighted, I usually wore contact lenses. Without either, I felt vulnerable, unable to read others' reactions, their body language. Putting the glasses on, I saw a room small and stark as a cell; bare, whitewashed walls broken only by one yellow-curtained window that looked out at the grey, full-bellied clouds as they moved swiftly past and away. The clouds were free. The window had no opening hinge. I wondered where they had brought me, but I wouldn't ask, nor enquire how long I'd been unconscious. Ignorance revealed leaves one's weaknesses exposed.[viii]

"Good morning, Clare. I am Sister Will. Nurse Bowden tells me you now are feeling better."

Anna Will was a big, blonde, Germanic woman. She uttered the word "better" with a gently teasing disbelief, implying that I could not possibly be truly feeling "better". I ignored it.

"Yes, thank you. Much better. I'm ready to go home."

Anna Will folded away her smile. "The doctors they will decide when you can go, Clare. In law you are underage. Until you are 21, you are without power to discharge yourself." I stared up at her in disbelief. Could I be imprisoned here, against my will, for two whole years?

"Never mind, my dear. I expect soon they will say you can leave." I gazed into the woman's square face and read there a wealth of kindness. "Today you stay in bed. Tomorrow you see Dr Fleminger.[ix] He will see how to help you. Now Nurse Bowden brings you more pillows and shows you where is the toilet and helps you later to have a bath. Then she sits with you, and you try to sleep." Automatically, Sister Will smoothed the white hospital sheet laid so neatly across my chest. Later I was to learn that, greatly respected by the doctors, Anna's no-nonsense approach prevented her patients from frightening themselves by losing control, while her own love of life permeated the ward atmosphere. I allowed a faint smile of acquiescence to twitch my lips. At least I wouldn't have to eat.

Not long afterwards Sister returned. "Clare, your mother has rung. She asks if you like her to visit?"

Her words sent my mind into reeling turmoil. My mother? My darling mother. How could I face her? And how would she endure seeing her "happy teenage daughter" in a psychiatric hospital, the very thing I had been trying to forestall? Our hometown, Haywards Heath, was dominated by St. Francis, a 19th century, eight-hundred-bed lunatic asylum, standing high and imposing on a slight rise behind the town. Whenever we returned home from the seaside or a walk on the South Downs, that asylum was the first sight to greet us; the last to fade into insignificance when we left. The place had featured prominently in ghoulish playground tales of madness.

I should have been dead, not lingering on. And now I would have to confront the guilt of causing my mother so much distress. It was then that I realised I was too much of a moral coward to meet her.

I turned to the sister and muttered, "No, not yet. When I get out. Then I'll see her. Not in here. She mustn't come here." And I turned my head away to hide my tears. Oh God, what had I done?

It must have been a couple of days later that I received the first of many letters from my mother, just like when I was at boarding school. Regular weekly letters, full of local news and chat. How my schoolgirl's heart used to sing at the sight of her clear, rounded writing on the envelopes, first, aged ten, at the Ursuline Convent in Belgium and then, through my teenage years, at an all-girls country boarding school in England. News of my brothers, my father and of course of all the innumerable things she was involved with in the community.

My mother was from that last generation of middle-class women who didn't go out to paid work but instead devoted themselves to running a home and supporting the local community. By this time she'd given up playing mixed field hockey with my father, but there were monthly teas and lectures that she organised for "Retired Gentlefolk", i.e. teachers and nurses and musicians. She loved driving and, unlike my father, was pretty good at it. She did Meals on Wheels and drove for the Red Cross, transporting the elderly to doctors' appointments. She was on a roster for flower arranging in our 12th-century village church and belonged to the ecumenical Wives Fellowship where, eventually, she became national president of the Senior Wives. She loved music and theatre and to play tennis—as a teenager she had played at Junior Wimbledon. No one expected Rosemary Thompson's daughter to end up in a psychiatric hospital.

Dave, too, wrote to me regularly; wise, comforting, encouraging letters. John and I, with six years between us, had never been so close. I was his 'little sister'. He was, by now, a married man with three small children and a demanding job to take care of. He restricted his brilliant, witty letters to Christmas, but they were always so well-crafted that each one was treasured. My father, too, was a busy man—and his handwriting was almost illegible.

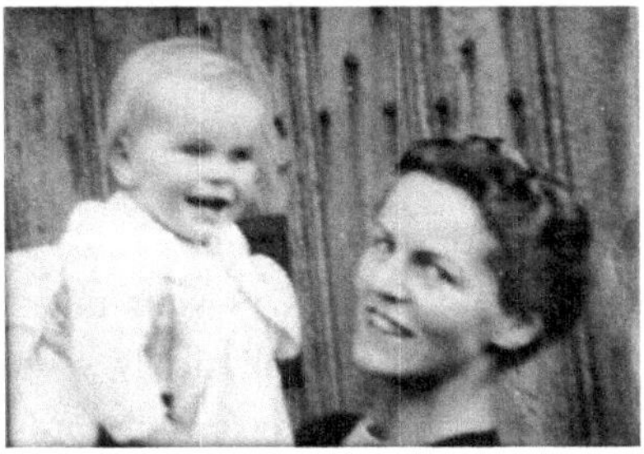

Clare as a baby with her mother Rosemary.

The next day I was summoned to meet Dr Fleminger. Nurse Bowden escorted me as far as the consulting room door, then left. Recently, I had developed an inexplicable fear of closed doors. Now my hand refused to grasp the handle as I battled with a petrified numbness paralysing my brain. In there I had to be alert and quick-witted.

Dear Lord, please tell them to set me free. It's my *life. They have no right to interfere.* But deep down I knew that my 'difference', my rejection of Life, cried out to society to be transformed.

Footsteps approached down the corridor forcing me to action. Fear made me knock too loudly yet I barely heard the brisk "Come in!" Dr Fleminger looked up from behind a large desk and briefly showed his teeth. *Why bother with words when it's so easy to judge a person by the sincerity of his smile?*

"Please sit down, Miss Thompson. This is Dr Christie, my registrar. He will be looking after you."[x]

I glanced quickly from one psychiatrist to the other. Dr Fleminger was a skinny man, almost as skinny as Mr Simons. Unbidden it came again, that green river of slime bursting down the old man's chest, slime which I couldn't stop. I shifted uneasily in my chair. Dr Fleminger spoke, but I didn't catch what he said.

"I'm sorry. What did you say?" Did my voice sound as strange and distant to them as it did to me?

"I asked whether you felt better."

"Oh. Yes. Yes, thank you." *Not too eager, not too vague.*

"The other day, did you mean to kill yourself?" His scepticism felt blatant.

"Yes."

The younger man sat forward. "Why did you want to commit suicide, Clare?" Dr Christie's voice, lilting as a caress, sent a shaft of warmth into my desolation.

"I didn't see it as suicide. I saw it as euthanasia. I couldn't stand the pain. Life had become one drawn-out pain."

Dr Fleminger cut in. "But it says in your notes that, once they'd operated, the surgeon found nothing physically wrong with you."

I looked down at my knees, searching for the words to explain. Then I looked at Dr Christie. "Does it really matter? I mean, I *feel* pain, whether you believe it's physical or not. My future is pain. People seem to think that one should go on living no matter what. I think that's crazy." My look defied Dr Christie to disagree. Instead, a smile lit his large brown eyes. I sensed the empathy, the spark between us. I liked him.

"So, you really wanted to die and just failed to do the job properly?" Dr Fleminger said.

"Yes. I messed it up."

"And now?"

The man wants to know what you are going to do now, Clare Thompson. What do you say? Grab the next opportunity to kill myself?

"All I need is something to stop the pain so I can sleep. Yesterday they gave me sleeping pills. I slept all night. I feel better already."

"Good. Well, Dr Christie will be seeing you three times a week. I recommend he sends you to pottery. Get that arm of yours working." Fleminger paused. "You may go, Miss Thompson."

I rose to my feet, clasped my blue dressing gown close around me. It made me feel naked, a body exposed on a beach where scavenging gulls come to peck sharply at the bones.

I didn't speak again as I left the office and returned to my room to plan.

"Clare! Up you get! Time to come and meet the other patients."

It was the next day. Nurse Bowden escorted me down the ward corridor to the day room. As we entered, a dozen patients looked up.

"Roland, this is Clare. Can she join you?" A wild-looking young man sporting a bushy ginger beard and single gold earring leaped up from the table.

"O-of course," he said with a broad grin and a mock bow. "W-w-welcome to the f-f-f-funny farm! Robert Gillespie Ward. Do you w-want to sit down? We're th-th-therapeutically engaged in d-doing a jigsaw." With a sweeping gesture he indicated the puzzle, the table, his companion. "Oh, and th-this is L-L-Lily. Lily m-meet Clare." The other patient, still in her dressing gown, looked up. I struggled to mask my shock. About my own age, she must have weighed 300 pounds or more. Lily squeezed up to make room for me at the table.

"Who are you under?" she asked by way of conversation.

"Dr Fleminger."

"Oh no, you poor cow! I'm lucky. I've got old Stafford-Clark.[xi] Quite a personality. Part of Penguin's defence team over the publication of *Lady Chatterley's Lover*. He's just written a definitive book called *Psychology for Students* and thank God, he's not a sadist." And Lily laughed, a brittle, street-wise laugh.

"I'm to see Dr Christie most of the time," I ventured, not wanting to be labelled a victim.

"Ah. Now you're talking. That's one gorgeous man! Watch out though. Everyone falls madly in love with him." She grinned mischievously at Roland. "They say Fleminger chose Christie on purpose. You know: first provoke the patient, bring out her anger, then leave her to turn with trustful confessions to Dr Big Eyes. Have you had a case conference yet?"

"No."

"Well, now there's a treat for you! It's Fleminger's *pièce de resistance*."

"Oh c-c-come off it Lily, you kn-know it's not that bad!" Roland cast an anxious glance in my direction."

As in the fleeting, unreal world of airport departure lounges or trains' railway carriages, so the here-today-gone-tomorrow atmosphere of acute psychiatric clinics encourages relationships to flourish, encourages people to share with strangers things they never dared share with anyone back home. In no time the three of us became close friends, annexing the unused patients' kitchen as our private den. It was these friends at the York Clinic who first showed me the value of talking therapy, of sharing.

Over the next two years it was predominantly patients, not staff, who eventually helped me. With them I sensed no judgement, no criticism, just a wish to understand. Maybe I misjudged the staff, the psychiatrists, maybe if I hadn't been so convinced that they were searching out my 'most grievous faults' I could have spoken to them too. Certainly, it was patients who gradually enabled me to heal, helped me to that distant goal of mental health, where each individual comes to accept themselves for who they are, faults and all.

Lily, Roland and I lived in an invisible bubble of trust as, determined not to be sucked into the system, institutionalised, I fought hard for my release.

"I don't know, Lily," I said a few days later. "I smile. I make my bed. Help lay the tables. Smile some more. What else do they want? I keep telling them I'm fine, that they can let me go, but it doesn't work."

"But of course not! You've got to use psychology to get out of this shit house. Their psychology. If you say you're better before they've even treated you, what's in it for them? Where's the ego trip? No. First you have to be 'sick', right. Pretend you've got some phobia or something. Then you have to allow them to 'cure' you. Then, hey presto, they'll let you go!" Lily glanced down at the glowing tip of her cigarette. "Do you feel like sharing why you're in here? Only if you want to. It sometimes helps." She wafted the question through the air, delicately, no more than the faintest flutter of an enquiry.

"Simple. I'm a failure. I failed to kill myself." I replied, equally lightly, dreading that Lily or Roland might pry further, but they didn't. They knew. According to the patients' code, even close friends never step unasked into that space where secrets lie hidden, but instead wait to be invited in.

"But th-that doesn't m-make you a failure, Clare. It just m-m-means you're not meant to d-die yet. It's your k-k-karma."

Lily interrupted Roland with a snort. "Karma! Don't talk karma to me. My karma stinks. I've been trying to escape it since I was 16." She turned to me. "That's when my dear, widowed father brought his tarty girlfriend into our home. You should see her, silly bitch." Lily waved her cigarette angrily. "She was always telling me what my father wanted. As if I didn't know! I'd looked after him for four years for Chrissakes! Oh yes, and she doesn't like young ladies swearing. It upsets her sensibilities." Lily flicked back the straight, black hair which kept slithering in front of her green, almond-shaped eyes.

Looking at her, I thought how stunning she would be—if only she could lose that excess flesh.

"So, Dad packed me off to The Cassel.[xii] You know, the world-famous psychiatric clinic for people with severe personality disorders, the place with great statistics for cures. God, it was ghastly. Everything was in groups: groups to cook, groups to wash up, groups to sweep the floors, clean the toilets, and then there was another, huge, group where we all sat around and discussed how each person had behaved in the first lot of groups. I refused. I'm not a sheep to be herded around in a flock. I'm a fucking individual."

I smiled encouragingly. I was beginning to feel proud of Lily's rebellion.

"Well, finally I'd had enough, you know what I mean." Her voice dropped to an embarrassed murmur, almost a plea. "I went to their dratted broom cupboard and shut myself in. Swallowed a bunch of sleeping pills I'd nicked from his pious mistress on my home leave the day before. I came round in hospital two days later. Of course, The Cassel wouldn't have me back after that. Oh God no!" Lily blew a contemptuous stream of smoke through her fine nostrils. "I was too much of a risk to their bloody statistics, wasn't I? Might have wrecked their recovery graph!" A bitter edge of rejection sharpened her voice.

In a flash I sensed an insight. As I sat gently rocking my aching arm, I realised that that was one of the good things about being inside. You seldom had to ask what others meant. In that ward, where the air hummed with tension, one quickly developed antennae that picked up the slightest nuance. Or maybe the antennae had always been there? Maybe that was what made us different: too thin-skinned, too intolerant of deception. I knew, just from her inflection, that Lily had only half wanted to die. Half had wanted to live or at least had wanted someone else to care if she did. Instead, she clearly felt both The Cassel and her father had rejected her. She had deliberately forced them to abandon her, at the same time hoping against hope that they wouldn't.

Bit by bit, I'd pieced together Roland's past. A young research scientist, in his spare time he'd experimented with drugs. Then one day something had gone horribly wrong, leading to his mental collapse. He had developed a stutter, lost his ability to do the simplest arithmetic and, with that, had lost his job. Yet he could still understand James Joyce. Soon he was feeding me with books, encouraging me to explore the poets Shelley and Browning and then to tackle Joyce's *Finnegan's Wake.*

Roland, like an older brother, took me under his wing. Unlike me, he had signed into the York Clinic of his own accord. He tried to persuade me that I, too, should co-operate. He couldn't see the point of me fighting them all the time. But he didn't understand. *He* didn't have something putrid fermenting inside him. Something that had to be kept hidden forever from all eyes, including my own.

One day I received a letter from Dave enclosing a copy of a note written by T.E. Lawrence to Bernard Shaw. It resonated deeply within me and, at our next get together on the abandoned kitchen's floor, I read it out to Roland and Lily.

"Listen to this. Do you remember I told you Dave's researching writing a possible biography of Lawrence of Arabia? He's just found this. It made me think of us. Me.

"Do you never do things because you must? Without wishing or daring to ask too deeply of yourself why you must? I just can't help it. You see, I'm all smash inside."

3

The Case Conference

THE KITCHEN DOOR swung open.

"Clare, time to get ready for your case conference."

My breath held in fear, I rose from the kitchen floor and left, refusing to meet the pity mixed with encouragement in my friends' eyes. Why, oh why wasn't I, like them, under Stafford-Clark?

As the nurse fussed round me, urging me to brush my hair, wash my face and tidy myself up, others were clearing the day room of all furniture except the chairs which were placed around the walls for the comfort of the spectators.

With the York Clinic attached to Guy's famous London teaching hospital, Dr Fleminger had no problem recruiting an audience from among its medical students. Backstage, we, his patients, were corralled in a small room already cluttered with the day room's tables. We stood silent, crammed and sweating.

"When's my turn?" I asked Nurse Peterson.

"That's up to the doctor, me lovey. Your job's to wait till you're called." Nurse Peterson treated us younger patients as substitutes for her own children who had long since flown the nest.

When all was ready, I watched through the half open door as Dr Fleminger came in procession down the ward corridor followed by his retinue in order of hierarchy: first Dr Christie, then the medical students, then, a little behind, Sister Will and the ward staff, with the student nurses bringing up the rear. The day room was large. Dr Fleminger took his special chair opposite the door. Christie and then Sister sat to one side of him while a chair reserved for the anxious client stood empty on the other. Thirty or so students filled the remaining seats.

As a patient emerged from the day room and shuffled towards the shelter of his bed, I wondered what they were discussing in there. Why did doctors abandon their famous code of confidentiality as soon as one was labelled mentally sick? Was it because this was part of a teaching hospital? Was that why, like exhibits in a freak show, we mental patients and our cases became almost public curiosities? Beneath my dressing gown, I could feel my nightdress sticking clammily to my armpits. I could smell my own fear. Any moment now I would enter that room watched by thirty pairs of eyes, eyes of students no older than myself, sitting in judgement on my sanity.

The door opened. A student nurse poked her head round. "Clare Thompson? Dr Fleminger will see you now."

I followed her into the arena, my arms clutched tightly across my chest as if to protect my soul. Just being in night clothes made me feel degraded, exposed. Dr Fleminger looked straight at me. I returned his gaze, praying he couldn't see my fear behind the mask of indifference.

"Good afternoon, Miss Thompson. Come and sit here. Tell us, Miss Thompson, do you have a university degree?"

My brain raced frantically from word to word. *Observe the use of 'us' just in case the audience had slipped my notice! Of course I don't have a degree. I'm 19, damn it! You didn't have a degree at 19 either. Anyway, you know I don't.*

"No." I forced the word out, flat and bored.

"Have you been to university at all?"

"No."

"Do you have any 'A' levels?" Somewhere nearby a medical student shifted uneasily. I switched my gaze away from the audience and stared at the door opposite.

"No."

"Ah! So, why is that?"

I let my eyes glaze over so I wouldn't see the medical students. But I couldn't stop the flush of mortification which suffused my face, nor the tears that pricked around my eyeballs. Dr Fleminger asked more questions, but I didn't reply. After all, he couldn't force me to. With any luck my silence in front of his troupe of students would embarrass him more than me.

"Well, if you have nothing more to say to us Miss Thompson, you may go."

* * *

"Clare, Dr Christie wants to see you."

I rose slowly from where I'd been lying on top of my bed, then paused to muster my defences. Dr Christie might prove harder to resist.

"Clare! Come on in!" His office was small but friendly. Books lined one wall and a tall window looked out onto the clinic's courtyard. But even here there was the ubiquitous 'sanity table' found in most psychiatrists' offices: one side for the staff, the other for the patient. A quite ordinary table put there to divide the sane from the insane—just in case either side became confused.

"So, how's the pottery?" Dr Christie smiled at me, relaxed, encouraging. I thought of the arrangement I had made one day with another patient and felt something warm, could it be pride, stir inside me. It had come to us simultaneously, in a gleeful flash as we stood in the Occupational Therapy Department. Paul had a gammy leg, the result of a near fatal car crash in his Jaguar, and I had my infernal arm. Our doctor believed both were psychosomatic and had sent us to pottery to force us to use our injured limbs. That day our joint efforts gave us exquisite gratification. As I pedalled the wheel, Paul, standing on his good leg, fashioned the wet clay with his good hands.

I have since discovered that just two years before I met him, Dr Fleminger published the findings of five years of research into hospital patient referrals to psychiatrists for undiagnosed pain.[xiii] According to his conclusions, 40% of patients had turned out to be suffering from hysteria or psychosomatic pain. Research by others around the same time showed that a shocking 70% of diagnoses of psychosomatic pain was made by male doctors against female patients. I was a teenage girl ripe for misdiagnosis and the humiliation of not being believed. Incorrectly, and almost fatally, I had been placed in this category which meant that, apart from anything else, I had to survive for months on end without painkillers, hardening my determination to kill myself as soon as I was released.

An operation some seven years later showed that my first neurosurgeon or, more probably, a junior registrar—had done a botched job leaving a splinter of bone behind, creating a lump of scar tissue that was crushing the nerve. The second neurosurgeon offered to give evidence in court if I wanted to sue the National Health Service over the pain, neglect and mental crisis I had suffered but, in the end, I couldn't face the stress.[xiv]

"Fine thanks," I replied to Christie's question. "Everything's fine."

"That's not what I hear from Sister Will."

Warily, my eyes flicked to his face. "What did she say?"

"That you cry out in the night. That you have nightmares which leave you white and shaking. Is that true?"

I paused but saw no way out. "Yes."

"Can you tell me about them?" He said the words softly, almost tenderly, as if luring a timid animal out of its hole.

I pushed back my hair and looked at him. "No, no I can't. Truly. I never remember. I just feel this unbearable terror. I can't breathe. I can't see. And then I wake up. Millions of people have nightmares. It's nothing."

"Are there any times when you're awake that you feel like that?"

"Only before a case conference!" I twisted my mouth into a cynical smile.

"Why do you fear those?"

"Why do I fear them? For a start, one has to open the closed door. I have a problem with closed doors. On the other side are all those people waiting to stare at you, the loony, as if you're some mutant with two heads. It's humiliating. You don't have to be mad to hate that, you know."

"No one's ever said you're mad, Clare."

"Haven't they? Then why am I here? Why won't you let me go?"

"Because Dr Fleminger's worried about you. You tried to kill yourself, remember? You were suicidal when you came in and we need to know why before we let you go."

"But I've told you and told you. I have this ruddy pain, and I couldn't sleep. Now that I take sleeping pills I feel better."

"But now you also have nightmares."

I took a deep breath. Was this perhaps the moment to 'get sick' as Lily had suggested? "Maybe it's something to do with patients dying. Maybe that gave me nightmares. I don't know."

"Did you enjoy nursing?"

"Yes, very much." And I smiled gently at the memory. I really had loved nursing. "When people got better. I enjoy looking after people. Only I was stupid. I never realised how many patients would die."

"How did it make you feel, when they died?"

"How did it make me feel? Guilty. A failure. Maybe even evil. You see, it was usually my favourite patients who died. It was as if being near me put a curse on them. The very first patient I chose to write a case history on died the day I handed in my report, the day he should have gone home. The first patient I 'specialed' died when I went to coffee. One night I went to help a friend during my lunch break. She was alone with a dying patient and was afraid. She'd never seen anyone die. I had. Half a dozen. Her patient's head was all skull with just a translucent film of skin stretched over it. Her wispy hair was a sort of defiant auburn. Maybe it was malnutrition, who knows? She was propped upright with lots of pillows. As I went round the screens she opened her eyes, eyes sunk deep with dying. She looked straight at me. Gasped. And died! Just like that. Just looking at me had killed her."

"Maybe there's something there for us to work on. We'll discuss it more next time." And he smiled at me, as he dismissed me. The session was over; as always, precise to the minute. I got up, smiled back and left.

*   *   *

I lay on my bed, gazing out at the scudding clouds, *Finnegan's Wake* open, face down, on my stomach. When Dr Christie had seen the Joyce on my locker he'd grinned.

"If you can get past page five of that you've a better brain than me." Christie had taken a degree in English Literature before switching to medicine.

I'd fought my way to page eight but, even with Roland's help, I was finding it heavy going.

Suddenly, the most glorious sound broke in upon my dreaming. Somewhere a woman was singing; pure, round notes full of melancholy. In here? Outside? I climbed off the bed and went to the window. No one. I opened the door. The sound grew louder. It filled the corridor. People had come out of the day room to listen.

"Ave Maria, gratia plena, Maria, gratia plena, Ave Dominus..."

Roland came up beside me. "Th-that's Sch-Schubert. It's Angela s-singing."

"I didn't know she could!"

"Oh y-yes. They say she was on her w-way to a gr-great future. It's the f-first time I've heard her sing in weeks."

"...mortis nostrae, et in hora mortis nostrae..."

As suddenly as it began the singing stopped, to be replaced by heart-rending sobs.

"Roland, she needs someone! Should I go in?"

"B-better you than me. She h-hates men."

"Will you open the door for me? Please!"

We went to the door and I knocked tentatively. "Angela, can you hear me? Can I come in?"

On the other side the weeping continued. I raised my voice. "Angela, I'm coming in. Okay?"

The sobs grew quieter. Roland opened the door, and I tiptoed through. Angela was lying face down, arms outstretched, crucified. I perched on the edge of the bed then put out a timid hand and touched her hair. "Angela, I had no idea you could sing like that. I wanted to cry too; it was so beautiful."

Angela rolled over and lifted a tear-stained face. "You mustn't call me Angela. My name is Gabriel. God told me. He told me my name is Gabriel. He sent me this." And she held up a silver medallion. "It's a gift from God."

"So is your voice, you lucky thing. Where did you learn to sing like that? Did you have special training?"

"God called me. He called me Gabriel. He gave me this medal. It's so I remember."

"So you remember what?"

For a moment Angela looked puzzled. Then she turned her back. "You have to go now. I need to speak to God."

I got off the bed and left.

"Roland, what am I going to do?" It was once again Thursday morning and I was sitting on the kitchen floor worrying at the quicks of my fingers, a habit I had acquired since admission. "I don't think I can survive another conference."

Roland was sitting beside me absently strumming his guitar. With his dancing eyes and gentle teasing manner, I had come to see him as my mentor, my wise advisor. Maybe more. Momentarily my thoughts shifted to something I'd hoped to casually find out about him for some time. I'd asked Lily but she didn't know either.

"Roland, can I ask you something?"

"Um-hum."

"Have you got a girlfriend?"

His strumming paused but only for a fleeting second. "I d-don't know, Clare. D-don't forget. I've l-lost my m-memory."

I digested this for a moment. "I never really understood that. How?" Instantly I flushed at my crassness, at stepping uninvited across the threshold of his inner space and hastily switched back to my own problems. "I'm sorry. Forget it. Maybe I should just refuse to go to the meeting? They can't physically force me."

"N-no, but you've got to be c-careful, love. You're under-age. There's n-nothing to stop them writing you up for E-ECT if they think it will 'h-help your treatment'."[xv]

I hugged my knees up under my chin and stared sombrely at the floor's black and white checked lino.

"It's criminal! How can we be so powerless? Electric shocks? Why not deep narcosis or go the whole hog and do a lobotomy, cut my brain in two? Can you imagine the fuss if doctors performed those on murderers or rapists? It's unthinkable. But on me, because I'm not 21, they can call it 'treatment', 'for the good of the patient'—and do whatever they bloody like." I was picking up Lily's defiant habits and rather enjoying them.

"At l-least deep-sleep tr-treatment's out. I've n-never heard of it being used here."[xvi]

"Roland, I've got to get out! They're driving me nuts. Look at me, sitting on the floor shredding my fingers!"

"C-Clare love, you've got to c-c-co-operate! You've got to h-help them to f-feel you're better. The longer you f-fight them the w-worse it will get, the more things they'll tr-tr-try out on you."

That afternoon I decided on a new strategy. I took out my contact lenses. Without them I could barely recognise my own hands, let alone all those people staring at me. It also boosted my morale to think I'd put one over on the doctor. And it worked.

The following week when I was summoned, I wiped my clammy hands down my dressing gown, pulled back my shoulders and made for the door. I had to go in quickly or he would know I was afraid. I grabbed and turned the handle, pushed the door open. Nauseous,

Head held high, I strode, unseeing, straight across the room to the patient's chair. Then froze. There was a blurred shape sitting in it. They'd changed the seating arrangements! Breaking into a sweat, I imagined creeping round the room peering blindly at each shape until finally I found the empty chair. It was Sister Will who came to my rescue. "Over here, Clare."

I was saved. Maybe Sister Will disliked the case conferences as much as we patients did.

A few days later I wrote again to David.

The York Clinic

Date unknown

Dearest Dave

So, the laugh was on me in the end, wasn't it? It wasn't the surgeon's dose that was wrong, but mine. Not enough pills to kill me. God, how I wish I was out of here. Oh, don't worry, Brother dearest, it's not bad in the widely imagined sense of a lunatic asylum; in fact it's highly middle-class and genteel: no raving, biting or frothing at the mouth. Everyone's far too scared someone might whisper that nasty little three letter word, 'mad'.

In fact, I've met some amazing people in here, indeed, some of the most intelligent people I've met in my whole life.

I keep telling myself, Dave, that I'm not psychotic, not schizophrenic, but what if they persuade me that I am? You remember how 'good' I was as a child? Happy, extrovert, but also 'good'? That was how others knew me—the good, happy one. That's who they thought I was. So that's who I became. It probably happens to everyone to a certain degree. Other people's labels help us to define ourselves. Maybe bad kids are bad partly because their parents and teachers keep telling them they are. And now I'm scared, Dave. Will I become 'mental' simply because enough people think I should be locked up?

Of course, they want to know about you and Mum and Pa and John but what is there to tell? Boy, how they'd relish hearing that I'd had an unhappy childhood! That I was beaten, degraded, sexually abused. Why, they'd swoop on it like vultures on a dead puppy. But I wasn't. We had a great childhood.

I didn't ask to be born, Dave. I owe no one my life. Indeed, I sometimes feel that I owe the world only my death. For the more I think about it the more certain I am that there *is* something evil inside me and I have to exterminate it.

But enough dearest bro. Do please keep writing when you have time.

And now, until I'm free dear Dave, adieu.

4

Testing! Testing!

THREE WEEKS AFTER my arrival, Dr Christie, sitting as usual in his office with me in the chair opposite, picked up the phone and asked for Nurse Bowden to be sent in. Then he turned to me. "I've organised for you to have some psychological tests, Rorschach and so on."

I flinched. I hadn't told a soul at the clinic about Dr Pinney, her tray of triangles and her findings. What might they not uncover now with their inkblots used, amongst other things, to diagnose schizophrenia, and their tests full of catch questions and hidden innuendoes?

Leaving the ward for the first time, I followed Nurse Bowden down to the reception area then along a corridor where she knocked on a door marked 'Miss E. Smyth. Psychologist'. Miss Smyth, in her late thirties, opened the door and showed me over to a diminutive table. It was a strange room, small and narrow. Intimate. Barely room for psychologist and patient to sit side by side.

"So, Clare, Dr Christie wants us to do some Rorschach tests. Have you heard of them?"

Panic! My heart started thumping hard. "Yes, but I've never seen one. They used to use them at the clinic where I worked." *To help diagnose schizophrenia.*

The 'inkblots' were actually meticulously hand-drawn by the Swiss psychologist Hermann Rorschach in 1921. He deliberately made each design as ambiguous as possible, leaving it open to a maximum number of interpretations. What people chose to see was somehow supposed to reveal their character. Recently, Rorschach's creations had become high fashion for personality assessment though their value remained fiercely contested. They were particularly popular when trying to treat patients who were reluctant to open up to their psychiatrists.

Miss Smyth held up ten, large, white cards, each about 7 by 10 inches, and waved them in my direction. "All you have to do is look at each picture as I hand it to you and tell me what you notice. You can turn it round, do what you like. As you can see, one half of every picture is basically the mirror image of the other, hence the inkblot label. As soon as you glimpse something, or more than one thing, just tell me what you see and where. No rush. Take your time."

Along with the inkblots went a special form where the test's administrator noted down each of the patient's moves under a code, a sort of shorthand to record the whole examination. Miss Smyth shifted her chair slightly away from my peripheral vision, slid the first inkblot along the table towards me, then picked up her clipboard and began swiftly filling out her annotated form, registering every one of my moves, hesitations, comments.

I felt the same anxiety that I'd felt months before when doing Dr Pinney's tests. Using the same caution, I studied the cards with great care. *So, this is what they look like. Nothing like what I'd imagined. Sharp-edged around the outside but much vaguer, more wishy-washy on the inside, somehow more sinister.*

"I see two disapproving foxes, with very pointed muzzles, facing in opposite directions." I heard Miss Smyth's pen scratching away. *So how do you interpret that? Is it what everyone sees? Am I somehow bizarre seeing foxes?*

Miss Smyth remained detached, sliding the next card across to me, trying not to impinge on my consciousness, leaving me to associate as freely as possible.

The next card seemed happier. "I see two elephants facing each other and touching their trunks together. They look friendly." Card four had something particularly disturbing about it. *Why do I feel it's horrible?* "I see a man on a motor bike, his body's huge and he's heading straight at me. Trying to kill me." But it was card number six that for a moment stopped me in my tracks. From the card's edge, a huge penis appeared, the urethra forming the midline of the two identical parts of the blot, with a small flower coming out of the tip. Confusion surged inside my head. *Why the fear? Come on Clare, you're a nurse! You've washed more penises than you can number. This is ridiculous!* A moment later pragmatism vanquished fear. My eyes cleared and I saw an even more obvious picture, that of an AK-47.

"I see an AK-47 with a flower coming out of the barrel."

Rorschach test over, Miss Smyth paused just long enough to hand me forms for a timed IQ test, then continued to calibrate my previous comments and her own observations. I settled more comfortably into my chair. I enjoyed the challenge of IQ tests: pitting my wits against 'theirs'.

At our next session, Dr Christie dropped my IQ results on the desk between us. "These," he said, "are a disgrace!"

I looked at him in astonishment. For once he actually sounded angry.

"How dare you abuse your intellect like that! These give you an IQ of 155, in the top one percentile of the population. Some people call that 'genius'. No wonder you're depressed! Why, with those results you could do almost anything."

"Surely that just proves how irrelevant IQ tests are?" I smiled sweetly up at him. "But wow! It's good to know I'm not plain stupid after all. So, I suppose that means I'm just lazy."

At first, I had found the handsome Dr Christie's warmth and intelligence both attractive and alarming, but I had discovered that without my co-operation, he was incapable of unravelling my inner terror, peeling away those precious, fragile, defensive layers; layers hiding I knew not what but something cataclysmically vile that no one must ever lay bare.

"Ah-hah! So that rankled, did it?" He raised an amused eyebrow. "Seriously, Clare, you should be at university or into journalism or something. Not messing around being a nurse."

"But maybe I like being a nurse." I chided him lightly.

He brushed it aside. "You've no right to waste your talent."

Abashed before his earnestness, I tried to explain. "You don't understand, Dr Christie. I really only have one talent and that is for IQ tests. And that's just a knack. Nothing else. I discovered it quite by accident."

The man smiled back. "You do yourself a grave injustice, young lady. You are also expert at tying our sessions up in knots, avoiding all discussion of your problems and generally defending yourself with your wits."

"Well now, isn't that a relief! All that IQ's not going to waste after all. So, what line of journalism had you in mind? Do you see me throwing new light on our psychiatric hospitals? Bringing understanding and insight to bear in interviews with lunatic psychiatrists?"

"Actually, Clare, I was thinking more of 'The Sewage and Garbage Collectors Weekly'." He looked seriously into my eyes, quenching at once my joy of battle as he alluded to my penchant for self-denigration and reminded me of our true relationship.

I was the first to look away.

As I left the room, I realised he hadn't mentioned the results of the Rorschach.

* * *

As Christmas approached, Sister Will galvanised everyone into decorating the ward corridor with paintings, cut-outs and acres of cotton wool. Sitting on the floor in the day room, cutting out pictures of the Three Kings, my thoughts drifted back to the family Christmases of my childhood.

Then I would sit on the playroom floor with my two older brothers, a coal fire burning in the grate, some craft work in my hands. In our household, Christmas was a time of creation: creating presents, decorations, cards. Very little was shop bought, for presents were thought to have less value if simply paid for. The labour was a labour of love, a gift from the heart. I diligently embroidered a tray cloth for my beloved great aunts, first selecting the design from transfers in my mother's embroidery box. These, placed face down on the white linen cloth, were then ironed on, leaving the faint blue lines of the floral design to be followed with needle and coloured thread. A handmade card with its Christmas greeting carefully penned inside was then slipped between the folds of cloth and the whole wrapped together, first in fine, rustling tissue paper and then in thick brown paper, tied up with raggedy string and sent off by post.

Thanks in part to all those Christmas presents, I learnt to love handicrafts in general. I remembered the fun Mum and I had in my mid-teens, driving down to Brighton by the sea to renew our summer wardrobes, spending hours together in the large fabric shop, first choosing three or four dress patterns out of the store's great stack of catalogues and then searching the bolts of cloth on the shelves for just the right materials to suit the outfits we had in mind, and finally selecting matching threads, buttons or zips. My mother cut and machined the dresses while, at the end, I sewed the hems with invisible, convent-taught stitching.

My main assignment, however, was knitting. I loved it. Away at boarding school, aged 12, I used to receive hanks of thick grey wool from the Mission to Seamen so I could knit them socks using four needles at a time. Next I got into fancy, multicoloured Fair Isle, Nordic and cable-knit sweaters. At the Belgium convent I'd learnt to knit Continental-style using the left index finger to put the wool around the needle. In England it was the right one that did the work. I soon discovered a way to have three different colours around three fingers of my right hand and another three on my left. I relished the challenge. Though one time my much older cousin bought skeins of expensive wool and asked me to knit her a beautiful Norwegian-patterned sweater. Something went disastrously wrong, and it finished up several sizes too large. I still feel bad about it.

Each Christmas at home there were new decorations to be made. Brightly coloured pictures, carefully reserved from magazines, were cut into strips and, using homemade flour glue and paint brushes, each of us would create lengths of chain, threading the next strip through the last link in the chain and then sticking the strips' ends together. Repeated over and over again, we'd end up with cheery paperchains to be strung right cross the playroom and the hall.

But for me, the real magic of Christmas was the tree. Our house had a staircase that curved up to the first floor leaving a well in the centre. On Christmas Eve, Dad would bring a large, freshly cut tree into the house and set it up in a bucket in the well. Not until we children were all in bed, did he start decorating it so that in the morning we could wake to its fairy-tale beauty: short, slender white candles in their silvery metal holders clipped on the tips of the branches and an exciting pile of presents stacked beneath.

In the York Clinic, I finished cutting out my Three Kings and took them out to the ward corridor to look for an appropriate space in the mural to attach them. Here, the idea of lit candles on a tree would have been met with horror. What, I wondered, would the rest of the family be doing now? Would they be gathering together around the fire? Would my absence cast a cold shadow over their celebrations? *Mea culpa! Mea culpa!*

All was finally ready for the Clinic's Christmas party. A time of false bonhomie, a time to remind many of dysfunctional childhoods, abusive parents, a fear of social failure, of exclusion. To add to the gloom, Roland and I were both on pills that forbade alcohol.

"Come on, Clare, I'm sure Mr Banajee'll let us have his sherry. He doesn't drink."

With just a few sips each, the alcohol instantly mixed with our medication, and we became almost falling down drunk, only managing to return to our ward by sitting on the floor of the lift and waiting for someone else to press the buttons.

Lily had been sent to spend the festivities with her father and his new wife. She came back screaming. "That fucking stupid bitch! I hate her! I'll kill her! I'll grind her into meatballs and barbeque her on a fucking skewer!"

They took her to her room and gave her an injection.

* * *

Days in psychiatric hospitals, presumably like those in prison, pass in soul-sapping sameness. Any physical demonstration of life in such places stands out as a landmark in the funeral march of time.

I was pacing up and down my room, digging my fingers into my elbow, trying in vain to force out the pain, when I glanced through the reinforced glass window to the courtyard below. There my gaze was caught by the sight of Angela. Angela with the voice of an angel, a genius for music—and an overpowering fear of men. Angela stripped naked, her dark hair trailing in black tendrils across her heavy white breasts.

She was backing warily towards the courtyard's exit, her body tensed, ready for flight. Two white-coated male nurses were closing in on her in a pincer movement, like hunters trying to corner a wounded deer. To anyone familiar with Angela's loathing of men, the sight was repugnant.

I went quickly in search of Nurse Peterson, the person we younger patients turned to in times of stress.

"Please, Nurse, it's Angela! She's in the courtyard. Trying to escape. Two men! They're trying to catch her. You know how she hates men. Please help her!" I could not suppress the quiver of anxiety in my own voice for I harboured a deep-seated fear that any request for help made me vulnerable to rejection.

Nurse Peterson gently touched my arm to reassure me, then left to see what she could do.

I returned to the window just in time to see Angela make a valiant dash for freedom. It must have been her consuming horror that sent her flying with such velocity down the drive and out into the main thoroughfare. Despite her size, the nurses, their white coats flapping like distracted gulls, were coming a poor second. I half-smiled as I imagined the housewives observing Angela from behind the safety of their net curtains, until finally some dreary, upright citizen, stiff-upper-lipped and blushing with embarrassment, would seize our Amazon of an hour and return her to her warders.

I thought of the degrading and inevitable return of the recaptured soul, caged once more behind invisible bars erected by a nervous society. A society that would not tolerate too much difference for fear that it might threaten its stability. I had not forgotten what Sister Will had said that first day, not forgotten that legally they could keep me captive for two long years until I, too, learnt to conform.

Despite several months in the Clinic, the idea that I might be diagnosed with schizophrenia still haunted me. After the Rorschach test, Dr

Christie should at least know if Dr Pinney had been right. At my next session I braced myself.

"Dr Christie, I want to ask you something." It came out all in a rush. He looked surprised. After all, it wasn't like me to be flustered or, for that matter, to ask questions.

"Anything you like. Fire away." He leant back, arms spread wide.

"Before I came here I was prescribed Neulactil. I looked it up. It's for schizophrenia. Am I schizophrenic?" I pushed my hair back in my nervousness.

"Schizophrenic! Of course you're not! Good God, why didn't you ask someone before? Why didn't you ask me?"

"I was afraid you'd say I was. You see I also met this woman, a psychotherapist. She said I would soon be schizophrenic."

"Said you'd be schizophrenic! What's her name?"

"Dr Pinney."

Dr Christie reached into the bookcase behind him and pulled out his copy of The Medical Register. He looked up 'Pinney'. Sure enough, the woman was there.

He grunted, then leant forward in his earnestness, his elbows resting on the 'sanity table'.

"Well, she's wrong. You're not schizophrenic. Okay, you've got problems—which, incidentally, you won't let us help you with—but that certainly isn't one of them and I'm quite sure Dr Fleminger would say the same."

"Thank you." I turned to gaze through the window. The evenings were stealthily drawing out. Winter had only a few hard weeks left to run. Spring with its hope of new life, its threat of new pain, was inexorably approaching. It was time I made my move.

"What are you thinking, Clare?"

With an effort of concentration, I forced myself to focus on Dr Christie, the judger of sanity, the gatekeeper to freedom—and death. I scraped together a vivacious smile and set it dancing.

"Nothing!"

For a moment his eyes danced in unison with mine. There was a definite spark between us.

"Liar!"

"Oh yes. Brazen."

"You know something, you're tough." We paused as each considered his statement, and from the pause I drew courage.

"Dr Christie, can you tell me something? When can I go? If I stay here much longer, I'll become ingrained in the kitchen's horrid lino."

"Just as soon as you're able to find yourself a job other than nursing, and to live a normal life again." I felt him scrutinising me. Was he searching for the infinitesimal stiffening of alarm which psychiatric patients often show when they are faced once more with the reality of the outside world? A world that had so recently rejected them or which they themselves had rejected. A world with which, due to some weakness in their own makeup, they were unable to cope. But in me I'm sure he saw no fear. I had never considered my stay in hospital as anything more than temporary. I had never inwardly allowed myself to be 'at home'. I had other plans and the first of these was devoted to being set free.

"Okay then, I'll go out and get a job tomorrow!" My voice sparkled, my pert smile dared him to try and stop me. He didn't. I think he had given up trying to unravel my problems. Without my cooperation we both knew it was impossible. Instead, he had been concentrating on persuading me to come to terms with life, to accept the difference between my often naïve ideals of human trust and kindness, and adult reality.

5

Outside

IN THE END, I didn't organise my discharge at all. Instead, Dr Christie contacted my parents, and they arranged for me to stay in London with close friends who found a job for me in the city's oldest bookshop, Hatchards, first opened in 1797.

Sitting in the Clinic's day room, a holdall at my feet, I waited nervously to leave.

The ward phone rang. Sister Will answered it and then walked over.

"That was Reception, Clare. Your mother she is waiting downstairs." She searched my face, her blue eyes anxious. I knew she cared. She'd always cared. She was a remarkable woman. She must have realised they were getting nowhere. Must have known, as I did, that the longer a person stayed inside one of their institutions the tougher it was to adjust to that other world, the harsh one outside the closed doors and windows that had protected them during their stay.

"Clare, I so hope things now will go better. That you will soon find life again outside. You can do it. I know you can. Sometimes patients they are afraid. Afraid they will fail. But you, I believe, are strong, my dear. You should not be afraid." And she put a compelling hand on my shoulder, as if willing her own confidence to flow across to replenish mine. I think she was maybe as confused about me as I was. For one day she would find my mind crystal clear and the next mysteriously mired in a labyrinthine tangle, snared on the borders of despair.

I smiled, looked Sister Will openly in the eye and thanked her. All the time I had been fighting for my release, it had never crossed my mind that, at my moment of victory, I would have regrets. Anna had been a good friend and mentor—even lent me Ayn Rand's *The Fountainhead,* with its message of putting your own happiness and achievements first and not sacrificing your life for others. I never converted to Rand's Objectivism, but I was grateful that Anna had tried to show me another way of looking at life.

Hastily I picked up my bag and headed for the lift. Then I hesitated and, on impulse, decided to take the two flights of stairs down to Reception. It gave me a few more minutes to muster the courage needed to face my mother.

In the last few days, since I had so brazenly told Christie I'd go out and find a job, I had begun, really for the first time, to examine the other consequences, the 'outside' consequences, of what I had tried to do four months before. Consequences I had barely considered during the inner chaos and pain that had led up to my attempted suicide, and which, unconsciously, I had refused to confront since. I had felt sure that killing myself was the only sane thing to do, the only solution. Best for everyone, not just me. Best for Mum and Dad too. What did the future hold for any of us? For me endless, grinding, demoralising pain and quite possibly madness; for them the possible shame of a lunatic daughter, and of being wrongfully labelled incompetent parents.

In all that time of planning, I had never once considered the possibility, or the consequences, of failure: that I could fail to die and end up in a madhouse. What if my parents hadn't understood that it was not only done for me but also for them? What if my own actions, my attempted suicide and then my refusal to see them in the Clinic had seemed, to my mother especially, like a cruel denial of our love for each other? Confronting these new truths, my sense of guilt grew until I was once again panicked at the thought of meeting her.

Before my admission there had always been such a close bond between us. Lying on my hospital bed, I had remembered fondly how, when I was a small child, Mum had read to me each evening in my bath. Her love of drama had brought the stories so alive that I almost believed I was inside the books themselves. First *Little Grey Rabbit* and the Beatrix Potter books. Then A. A. Milne's *Winnie-the-Pooh*, and the enchanted poems wrapped in his anthology *When We Were Very Young*. How I had loved the puppy who'd gone 'up in the hills to roll and play'. And how I'd shivered at the thought of the bears waiting to pounce in *Lines and Squares*. Next had come the Edwardian tear jerkers: *The Secret Garden, A Little Princess, What Katy Did* by which time I could read perfectly well on my own but enjoyed the books much more when my mother's voice brought them so evocatively alive. I must have been seven or eight when, late one night, Mum had come storming into my bedroom demanding to know what I thought I was doing with the light still on.

"I-I-I'm reading Heiiiiidi!" I wailed. I'd just arrived at the climax of the young heroine's misfortunes.

Ever pragmatic, Mum's face softened. "Well then, you'd better finish it, hadn't you?" And she'd walked out, closing the door gently behind her.

As I reached my mid-teens, the two of us had shared so many delights: visits to the theatre, music, playing tennis on the sunken, weedy grass court in our rambling garden.

It was usually in late spring that 'Operation Marking Out the Tennis Court' began. First, we got out the ancient lawnmower that made a clacketty-clack sound as you pushed it over the grass. Once the cuttings were dumped on the compost heap, we went round the lawn with metal skewers, probing down through the earth where we thought the metal 'corners' of the white-lined court should be. Over the winter, these metal right angles had sunk beneath the grass. Then, the eureka moment as skewer clinked on metal, and we prised one up. The court had a distinctly soggy attitude, with quite a dip just beyond the back line where my father said an underground stream ran. Knowing the uneven terrain certainly gave us a home advantage.

Next came the best part. Out of the potting shed came another ancient contraption into which Dad mixed a sort of plaster and water-based white paint. Armed with a very long piece of string with a skewer at each end, we'd stretch the string taut from one metal corner to the next. Whoever was in charge would then carefully guide the roller along the string. Hey presto, the first white line! Sadly, being the youngest, I seldom got a chance to have a go.

Now, I paused at the final bend in the stairs to look down, unseen, on my mother. Was it my imagination, my guilt, or did she already look older, diminished? Was her softly permed brown hair turning grey, her fine features more wrinkled, the angle of her head somehow a little less compelling? A wave of love and regret swept through me as I hastened down the last few steps, dropped my holdall on the floor and ran to enfold her tightly in my arms. Always so much smaller than me, I suddenly felt a keen protective love for her and wondered why I had been so afraid of meeting her, so ashamed that I had asked Sister Will to tell the family not to visit. Was it really guilt I felt? Or was it this inexplicable sensation that I had of some unknown degradation, some vile poison that lurked somewhere deep inside me, not to be shared with anyone and, above all, not with my mother?

It seemed strange to find spring putting forth its first green shoots outside the centrally heated walls of my jail. As I carried my holdall out towards the waiting taxi, I finally knew a flicker of fear. What had I done, and what was I going to do now? Involuntarily I glanced back and saw for the first time the outside facade of the York Clinic, the place that I had entered unconscious on a stretcher and where I had lived for the past four months or so. I saw the warmly lit entrance hall, the womb that had sheltered me, had allowed me to suspend for a while a final decision on my future. I had forced this parturition myself, and so I had, once again, to struggle for life in the cold.

The drive through the London traffic to the flat of my oldest friend, Sue,[xvii] challenged both my mother and me. After that initial embrace, I sat, backed into one corner of the cab, wondering how to break the silence, how to reconnect to the mother I had always loved, how to start to repair the damage my attempted suicide must have caused.

My mother, meanwhile, sat beside me no doubt worrying anxiously whether it would be best to speak or to keep silent.

A reserved, discreet woman, my mother had been lovingly reared by her aunts, while her father, a Scottish doctor, worked with the British Army in India accompanied by her mother. Just after the First World

War, it was considered by many to be too dangerous for European children to live in India for fear of sickness: plague, leprosy, malaria, cholera. So, my mother, Ro, and her brother, Norman, were cared for by relatives back home; her brother with their maternal grandparents and Ro with her mother's three unmarried sisters—my beloved great-aunts, Fuff, Timmy and Gee.[xviii] It was a gentle household which formed my mother's character. Fuff was a blue-stocking, Timmy taught my mother at Wimbledon High School and Gee founded one of Britain's first physiotherapy schools at Kings Hospital, London.

Finally, in the taxi, in a strained, self-conscious voice, I said, "Thank you for all your letters, Mum. They made such a difference. And thank you for fixing things up with Sue. Do you think she minds me staying?"

"No, not at all darling. She seemed fine about it. Of course, you should pay board and lodging once you receive your first wages." Then my mother took my hand and patted it affectionately.

"Mummy, I'm so sorry about all this," I rushed on. "It was the pain. That man saying I would have it for the rest of my life. And then writing me up for pills for schizophrenia. I just couldn't face it. You do know that it was never against you and Daddy? It was more to save you from shame, shame of having a mad daughter. But instead, I seem to have brought you more humiliation."

Mum squeezed my hand tightly where it now lay on the leather seat between us. "There now, let's not talk about it. That's all in the past. I think you'll love working in Hatchards, don't you?"

So that was that.

Sue Pick and I were life-long friends. Our mothers had done everything together: tennis, mixed hockey, Wives Fellowship meetings, Fine Arts lectures. We had drifted apart as we went to different boarding schools and took up different careers, but now, together in the Pick's London flat, in no time we were wallowing in reminiscences. Mrs. F, our outsized, kindly babysitter, had featured large in our early childhood.

"Do you remember doing back-to-backs in the bath?"

"Of course!" I laughed. "You'd stretch your legs out straight pushing against your end of the bath, forcing me to bend my knees up tight at the other."

"And then you'd straighten your legs out full force," said Sue, "And we'd get into a great rhythm sliding up and down until we built up a tidal wave. Water everywhere!"

"And do you remember the time poor Mrs F got really cross? After all, she was the one who was going to have to mop up the mess, but we didn't think of that aged four and five. That time she came in and said, 'If you go on doing that, when you die you won't stay in Heaven but come back to earth again, and you won't come back as a nice dog like Moony, you'll come back as nasty insects!"

Hatchards was large and it was posh. One day, writing out a receipt for a beautifully turned out, middle-aged, customer, I asked for her name. She replied, "Princess..."

I had taken the job to keep my promise to Dr Christie: to give Life a chance. I worked hard, tried to greet customers cheerfully and was soon being congratulated on my sales. But that only added to my misery. I loathed that label of competence and responsibility, the stress of always aspiring to perfection—and always failing. And yet I sought it out. That was my identity. That was who they said Clare Thompson was. With each passing day I felt more trapped, more wretched, out of control, like a cable car whose brakes have failed, careering downwards on an inevitable course towards obliteration.

Travelling home from work one day, I found everything somehow more finely etched, more detailed, more irritating. I looked in the smart shop windows at their rows of mannequins, all simpering smiles and purple nails, displaying the latest fashion, a fashion followed slavishly by the sheep who hurried past. *And next year they will all be wearing something different because some designer has said that that is what people should wear. And half the globe is starving. And you, naive little misfit, actually had the arrogance to think that you could do something about it. You thought that you were going to go out and save the world. Huh! And all you did was sit there while your patients died!*

I watched as buses, taxis and cars jostled for position in the endless crawl towards distant death. The drivers, their faces tense, waited to pounce on the chance to get half a wheel ahead of the next man, poised to sound their horns with pent up anger if the move was frustrated. What was the point? They were all going to die sometime. The gutters were choked with litter and cigarette butts. Yet society didn't condemn as insane anyone who tried to smoke themselves to death—provided they claimed at the same time to love Life. Only if a person honestly rejected it as pointless did society seek revenge.

I arrived back at the flat totally exhausted by the chaos within; the physical pain, the night terrors, the dread of madness, and now the old fear of closed doors swelling up out of control and taking over my mind. There were so many doors to negotiate: the flat door, the shop door, the lavatory door. Each had to be faced with the same stomach-squelching tension that others reserved for a major interview. And each one wore away at my resolve to give Life a chance.

Things finally came to a head, was it after a month or six weeks? Sue was trying to encourage me to join her and some friends on a trip to the cinema. "Come on, do! The more you shut yourself away, the more cut off you're going to be."

"No, you go on. I'll be fine. I'm really tired."

"OK. Suit yourself!" Sue shrugged and got up. She'd tried. What else could she do?

It was OK for her. She was everything that a young Sixties woman was supposed to be: fun, confident, pretty, petite, a popular party goer, head of sports at her boarding school. For a while in her junior tennis days she'd partnered the British tennis player, David Lloyd.

After Sue went out, I sat for a while reflecting on boyfriends. Mine were all like me: second division. There was the Indian accountant whom I let down. A Polish artist who tried to get me onto hard drugs. An older man who claimed to have the first Mark X Jag in London. The only one I really cared for was Simon. Indeed, I was crazy about him, but then he moved on and I was left, defeated, to sing that folk song, over and over again, the one that goes, "Once I had a sweetheart and now I have none. He's gone and leave me to sorrow and mourn."

I sat for many minutes without moving; my eyes staring blank and empty into the far corner of the kitchen. *You'll never get better. You know that. There's a huge snake of evil coiled up in your belly. It's feeding off the green slime that's inside you. What are you waiting for? Till everyone knows whatever it is that you've done? Till Mum and Dad are publicly humiliated? Why wait? Why suffer? Just a short while and it will all be over, the pain finally gone.* It was as if I had been marking time, building up my strength both mental and physical for another assault, marshalling my energy for the next attempt to wipe myself out.

I went to my room and lay down, fully clothed on the bed, my eyes open, staring into the darkness.

The following day I travelled to work in a daze. I looked neither right nor left as I crossed busy thoroughfares as I had lost all fear of cars. I barely heard the brakes squealing or the drivers shouting at me and hooting. If a car got me so much the better. I didn't think of the drivers or my parents at all.

I spent much of the morning in the staff rest room before telling the supervisor I was unwell. Then I went to the Natural History section and carefully selected a large and beautiful book on trees, symbol of Life. I bought it at staff discount from the head cashier and then had it gift-wrapped. I re-read the letter I had written in the early hours of that morning.

Dear Dr Christie,

This is just to say thank you for trying to help me. I'm sorry I've let you down. But you know, I wasn't worth the trouble. I did try. To give Life a chance, I mean. But I was not strong and healthy and brave like the trees. I was a green river of slime, hypocritical and death-giving. Don't feel sad when you see this. I'm not. Just relieved that at last the charade is over. And that the pain, the pain that no one believes in, will finally have stopped. My life was but an invisible mote in the eye of Time. My death will change nothing. Except to wash away my contagion.

'The ploughman shall go out in March and turn the same earth
He has turned before; the bird shall sing the same song.'
T.S. Eliot, as I'm sure you know.
Yours sincerely and with thanks
Clare

I folded it and tucked it into the wrapping paper. It was odd to think that I, Clare Thompson, would no longer exist when he opened it. I left the present with the postal department and went out into the street.

In order to avoid suspicion, I had decided to visit three chemists in turn. I was not certain of the lethal dose of Aspirin, it was not one of the things they taught in nurses' training, but I had read of an empty bottle found beside a corpse so decided to go beyond that and added a bottle of Codeine. Four cartons of Kia-Ora orange drink completed the list. With all the purchases in a large paper bag, I went into the Oxford Street News Theatre.

Originally, I'd thought of dying in the flat but that seemed grossly unfair on Sue. The next possibility was a public lavatory but, during a practice run, I had been disturbed within ten minutes by someone rattling at the handle to see if I was alright.

The idea of a News Theatre had come to me some days ago, based on the theory that one is most alone in a crowd. *Obviously it's no good keeling over in the fountain in Trafalgar Square. Some busybody's bound to think you've had an accident and fish you out. No, the News Theatre is the place, with people coming and going all day and vagrants sitting there in the dark for hours just to warm up. Provided I slouch in my seat and don't collapse into a neighbour's lap, I should get away with it.*

Just the fact of my preparations had already raised my spirits.

It took several minutes to get used to the darkness inside the cinema. I looked about me, hesitating, weighing up between a seat on its own or one beside others where, from a distance, I would be less conspicuous. The usherette's torch wove its way in my direction and bade me follow.

The small, round circle of light led towards the back of the cinema and to one side. I quietly slipped from its imperious beam into a row near the lavatories, leaving three vacant seats between me and the aisle.

I sat for a moment considering my next move. The darkness was confusing. I had overlooked the problem of choosing a seat.

Once I'd collected my wits, I went unobtrusively to the illuminated 'TOILETS' sign. Steeling myself yet again, I pushed open the door and branched right for the Ladies. Entering one of the cubicles, I placed the paper bag on the floor. It was hard to distinguish it in the feeble light seeping over the door. It was harder still to swallow the pills. I started with the Aspirin, pouring them out in handfuls and cramming them into my mouth. I had to suck up enough juice through a straw to lift the dry, clinging pills off my tongue and down my throat. In the end I discarded the straw and poked a large hole in the carton with my latch key. I paused before unscrewing the cap of the Codeine bottle. The pills were so big my courage almost failed me. Now I could only take a few at a time and I was already awash with Kia-Ora.

Abruptly, a jet of bitterness spewed from my mouth into the lavatory pan. On my knees on the grimy tiles, I clutched the sides of the enamelled bowl, begging my stomach to stand firm with the rest and not ruin everything with such an unnecessary display of weakness. Peering down into the bowl, I tried to estimate how many pills had been lost. I had only vomited once. Maybe it was just the Codeine which had returned. The acrid smell made my pull away and stand up, my back against the door.

I waited perhaps another three minutes, completely still with eyes closed, till all feelings of imminent gagging had passed. Then I cautiously pulled the chain and moved very gently towards the door so as not to disturb the precious load I was carrying, like a foetus of death, in my belly. It was my own creation, my own solution to a paltry life gone wrong.

I deposited the rest of the Codeine plus the empty bottles and cartons in the rubbish bin and then made my way back to settle myself low in my seat. There was no one else in the row to want to climb out and, slouched as I was, it was unlikely that anyone would try to climb in. I relaxed and waited to die.

An hour later I was still waiting. *Those reports in the papers were misleading. '... a half empty bottle of Aspirin was found beside the bed...' They never say how long the corpse had waited to die. Obviously not just half an hour! God, and I've always loathed cartoon films. What the hell made me choose a News Theatre?* I couldn't even remember if it was the second or third repeat of the programme.

I shifted my weight gingerly so as not to aggravate my insides and yet relieve the numbness that my strange contortions had produced in my buttocks. An usherette stopped and asked if I was all right. I turned and smiled whitely into the torchlight, nodded and replied truthfully, "Fine, thank you."

Another hour and then another passed, and I could still find no signs of death in me; no dizziness or faintness, just a high-pitched ringing in my ears and a dry, hot flush to my cheeks. Then, without warning, a great wave of nausea swept over me, and I had to dash headlong to the lavatory. There my stomach heaved and heaved. No individual pills now, just white grit and foam. I tried to halt the exodus, but it just came on and on, in great body-shuddering bouts and I cursed feebly at the sight of it all, and at my helplessness and hopelessness. And then I burst into tears.

As soon as the worst had worn off, I left the cinema and groped my way outside. I was stunned to find that the sun was still shining on the pavement, that the whole world had not gone dark in mourning for my failure. Then another attack gripped me, and I puked into the gutter.

Feeling utterly despicable, vomiting in front of crowds of shoppers, I dived in shame for the Oxford Circus Underground. But as I walked hastily down one of the long tunnels to the ticket office, I was sick again. This time there was no gutter. Would someone clear up the mess before the rush hour? I imagined a great pool of vomit trampled by unseeing feet, felt the soft squelch as the feet subsided into it and trailed my cloying degradation after them. I fled again in revulsion to the fresh air.

The taxi pulled over almost at once, but where to go? I gave the address of the flat and, as the cab edged out into the traffic, was sick once more, this time out of the cab window. I vomited three times in all before we reached our destination. By then I could barely muster the energy to pay the driver or fit my key into the front door.

When Sue returned from work, I was lying semi-comatose on the sofa.

"I'm terribly sorry, Sue, but I think you better get me to a hospital."

6

Electro-Convulsive Therapy

MIDNIGHT WAS APPROACHING by the time they wheeled me upstairs, all signs of white grit pumped out of my stomach. In the ward the lights were dimmed except around the first bed. Glimpsing the woman's yellowing face and sunken eyes, I knew at once that its occupant was dying.

Sclerosis of the liver I thought absently as they wheeled me past. *Why do they all die except me?*

They put me into the next bed, pulled the curtains around me and turned on the overhead lamp. A young houseman came in to check my vital signs: blood pressure, pulse, temperature and respirations. By squinting down my nose and flipping the thermometer in my mouth up with my tongue, I could just read 106° F.

Well, you're still in there with a slight chance, girl. Maybe Aspirin burns you up like hell fire. The thought had barely found time to settle before the doctor turned to me.

"Well, you're not going to die this time." The words came with an upbeat emphasis though underneath he must have felt bitter for, as he struggled in vain to save the life of my neighbour, so he was also obliged to spend time keeping a life-vandal breathing.

"Have you got ringing in your ears?"

"Yes." My voice, coming from far away, superimposed itself on the noises in my head.

He listened to my lungs, palpated my abdomen. "Where do you live?" His voice was kinder now. Maybe he'd decided I must be sick too—in my head.

"I don't remember." It was of course a lie, but they couldn't prove it. The doctors downstairs had promised to discharge me the next day. I had made them promise before I agreed to spend a night in the ward. The last thing I wanted, now that I was still alive, was for my parents to find out.

From nowhere came the memory of my father's embarrassed words, "You do know don't you, that if you succeed in killing yourself, it will kill your mother." For my dear, introverted father, that was quite a statement; one I had forced myself to forget in the past weeks of obsessive planning. By now I was half convinced that inside me I was harbouring something so evil that it could destroy the whole world. A great wash of misery rose and broke unheard inside my skull. I waited for tears, but no tears came; guilt, self-pity, self-loathing and despair fused in silent communion. My skin burned dry with fever, the muscle that was my heart fluttered timidly, unwanted in my chest. I caught my breath in deep gusts. I was still alive... and all alone. I had failed again. I listened to the intermittent, rasping breath of the patient in the next bed. *She'll be dead by morning.*

As dawn broke through the ward windows, I woke and saw that the neighbouring bed was empty. Pristine white linen waited innocently to offer succour to the sick. The ringing had faded from my ears till it formed only a backdrop instead of the main orchestration. The burning was dying from my cheeks. My body was damp and exhausted.

On the ward, clean-starched aprons relieved limp creased ones. The day sister came over and took my pulse.

"That's better, dear. Your parents phoned last night. They were worried about you." Reproach lurked in the sister's voice. Probably she, too, was a mother. "The doctors say you can be discharged later." I hardly heard the last words as guilt swooped down.

About mid-morning two orderlies with a wheelchair stopped at the sister's desk. After a short consultation, she pointed to my bed and led the escort over.

"Here we are then, Clare. These two gentlemen have come *to take you away.*"

I listened only to her tone, wondering why people so often talked to me as if I were mentally defective or a small child to be humoured. Then her meaning penetrated. To take you away.

"Where are they taking me? You said I could be discharged!"

I sat up rigid in bed, trying to control the terror. A voice was screaming in my head, *Don't let them know you're afraid! It'll give them power, power to wipe out your identity!*

"You can't expect us to send you back to your flat after what you've done! We're discharging you to the York Clinic." Sister's tone turned aggressive as she defended her deceit. That aggression in turn gave me courage to fight back.

"I'm not going! You've no right! You said I could go home." My voice hissed out, venomous with fury. "You lied to me, God damn you, you lied!"

One of the men stepped forward and took my arm. "Come on lass, nothing to get upset about."

I spun round. "Don't you touch me! Take your hands off!" In my mind's eye I saw Angela, that poor, trapped spirit making a desperate bid for freedom. I raised my voice louder, "I'm not going there! You can't make me. Let go of me, you, or I'll scream!"

The man looked uncertainly at Sister who gave a scarcely perceptible nod. My arm was released. Sister moved closer and took both my hands firmly in her own. From being domineering she became gently understanding.

"Clare, love, you mustn't be afraid. You almost died last night. We can't let you out on the street now, you're not well. The York Clinic wants to help you. We have to send you there. You know that. Getting upset only makes things worse. Would you perhaps like an injection to help you?"

The sister's soothing tones quenched my vibrant anger. I felt my body shrink away to nothing. My eyes turned darkly in upon myself as the threat of an injection forced me to co-operate. Like Angela I was trapped with no place to hide. Shaking my head, I stepped slowly down and into the wheelchair. Sister wrapped a blanket around me, patted my back, and handed my notes and a plastic bag of my street clothes to one of the attendants. Around the ward the other patients returned to their morning papers and their knitting, reassured that order had been restored.

Numb. Numbed body and soul by the return. I had been so sure that this time I would die. Did I have the energy left to fight again for my release? To fight the fine mesh of psychotherapeutic interpretations, the institution of insanity itself?

I lay staring at the wall, ignoring all efforts to rouse me. For what? The feeling of emptiness, of desolation was complete, my spirit burnt out.

"Sit up, Clare. Here's Dr Fleminger to see you." Sister Will's voice was troubled. Did instinct tell her that this time I'd moved much closer to the brink? I remained quite still, facing the wall. I was not there in my body. I had left it, to float where none could lay hands on me or wrench me from my safety, detached and unmoved above the pandemonium of my life.

Dr Fleminger spoke. "Back again Miss Thompson? I'm afraid you betrayed our trust, didn't you?" He paused but received no response as I listened from far away. "I've told Sister to see that you have a nurse with you 24 hours a day. If you wish to go to the toilet you must leave the door open so the nurse can watch you, keep you under surveillance at all times." Sentence passed, the doctor left.

A nurse took up position on a chair near the door.

* * *

I must have drifted in limbo for more than a week while my bruised and battered spirit slowly resurfaced. The hospital's broken promise not to tell my parents, their lie in telling me I'd be discharged, combined with the weight of my own guilt, my failure, all added to make me feel even less sure of myself and my sanity.

One morning I was given a shake by the nurse on guard.

"Clare! Wake up! Here's Dr Christie."

Dr Christie walked breezily into the room, dismissed the nurse and looked at me for a moment as I lay in the high hospital bed.

"Hello Clare." He paused to allow his soft, velvet voice to carry its magic past my vacant mask. How long, I wondered, had he spent cultivating that reassuring voice. "Not so good, I hear." He watched my face. Was he looking to see if I was as withdrawn as the staff reported?

"I must thank you for the book. It's very beautiful." He spoke almost lovingly, his voice warm with compassion. "You thought you'd be dead when I got it didn't you, poor old thing?" And he placed a consoling hand on my wrist. Instantly I stiffened. Fear screamed out, wrenching apart the comforting fog of my withdrawal.

Dr Christie removed his hand. "Clare, do you know why you hate so much to be touched? Can you tell me? Does it have something to do with why you need to destroy yourself?" His voice barely rippled the silence. I turned my eyes away from his but gradually a memory returned of that conviction and despair that had driven me on. Perhaps I should tell this man, perhaps he would understand.

"I had to do it." The words came husky and laboured, my voice creaking from disuse. "I have to die. Can you understand? It's my duty. I'm evil. I'm in pain. And now I think I'm going mad." There, I'd said it. Let them find something worth living for in that litany.

"How do you feel right now?"

I could have said "fine" as before but they would not believe me, and anyway I felt too tired to fence with them. At least if I said "lousy" they might leave me alone. As Lily had once said, 'They're always happy to believe you—provided you agree you've got something wrong!"

Dr Christie waited. Silent.

"I feel lousy." I mumbled, keeping my face averted, ashamed that they had won even that small victory.

"Okay old thing, I'll write you up for some tablets. They should make you feel a bit more cheerful. I hope you'll soon be well enough for us to get rid of your special nurse. Meanwhile, I'll send her back in."

With the return from limbo, the full indignity of my position struck home. My freedom confiscated, I wondered how the staff would face the mortification of being watched twenty-four hours a day, lavatory and all, where passing patients could view me through the open door. Grey limbo beckoned. I now returned there often, my only hiding place. As I drifted free from my body, I knew no one could touch me, nor diagnose, nor probe.

*   *   *

Two days later Dr Christie came again.

"Good morning, Clare. How's things?"

"All right."

"Hmm. I don't believe you really mean that. But do you think you are making some progress this time?" I gave a shrug of indifference. Who cared? What to him was progress was to me a betrayal of my beliefs.

He took up his favourite position perched on the end of the bed, one foot touching the floor, the other swinging free. Absently he picked at the bedspread. For a moment I felt my eyes soften. Christie was always generous enough to reveal a little of his humanity.

"The staff are worried about you, Clare. We feel we aren't helping. You still seem pretty depressed." He looked at me, searching. Did instinct tell him that only honesty would reach me? I replied with a blank mask, too tired, too depressed to care. He sighed. "We were wondering how you would feel about having some ECT to see if that might help you." He hesitated for I'd come to life, chin up in preparation for a fight. "Your parents have signed the form."[xix]

There they go again. They had me trapped. Bound fast to do their bidding for eighteen more mind-destroying months. Was this a punishment to me for coming back? I didn't blame my parents. I'm sure they believed, or at least hoped, the doctors were doing the best for their daughter. They were bewildered, felt overwhelmed, wanting to do all in their power to help. After all, the doctors were the experts. In my parents' place I would almost certainly have done the same.

"Frightened?" Dr Christie asked with his questioning, winsome smile. Still my chin stayed up as I stared past him, expressionless.

"No. I'm not afraid of electro-convulsive therapy." And it was true. I liked to use its proper name, especially to the staff. ECT or treatment or shock treatment were all pallid euphemisms, and therefore more comfortable, beside the resonance of "electro-convulsive therapy"; all ways to disguise the fact that doctors intentionally gave patients epileptic fits by passing electric volts through their brains. No one knew why it was beneficial but, in selected cases, ECT did indeed work miracles.

"Good. Well, we'll see how it goes, okay? We'll start tomorrow morning.

Sister will tell you what to do." Dr Christie went briskly out of the room to be replaced at once by the special nurse who glanced knowingly at me before returning to her sentry post by the door.

So, everyone knows already. Dr Christie had merely performed a charade of seeking my agreement as they expertly shifted the pawn across the board.

Next morning I had no breakfast. Instead, I lay as instructed on top of my bed, my head at the foot, waiting for the machine to be rolled in. Were they perhaps going to use a guillotine? As the footsteps approached, I felt a slight quickening of my heartbeat but whether from excitement or apprehension I couldn't tell.

"Hello Clare. I'm told this is your first treatment. Is that right?" I looked at the anaesthetist in wonder as he deftly wrapped a tourniquet round my upper arm. He actually sounded as if he expected me to make a normal reply, to be a normal human being, in no way inferior or defective or to be humoured! He placed a small cylinder of wood in my hand.

"Could you grip on this for me?" It was excitement, not fear, that ran through my veins. A challenge from the unknown, a new experience in the unutterably dreary round of nothing which was my daily existence. The sharp reality of ECT was helping my zombied self to come alive. The doctor massaged my arm firmly, bringing up the vein.

"Now, I'm going to give you a prick and then you'll go to sleep."

Just a little prick. The words reverberated from my childhood, that time when I had been seriously ill. At first, they had not believed in that pain either, implied that I was making it up, lying. How I hated them for that. I was in agony. A sample of black urine put paid to their disbelief. Then they had given me anaesthetic after anaesthetic as they probed and searched, trying to find out what was wrong. They finally understood my excruciating pain when they uncovered a benign tumour almost completely blocking the tube from my kidney to my bladder. An unheard-of phenomenon, it had been written up in the British and American Medical Journals. But always they fed me the same demeaning lie, "Just a little prick, dear!" The child in me had rebelled and the anaesthetist had learnt to say, "Now for the big jab!" The nurses had not approved, but how I had loved him for his honesty, for the dignity of his acceptance of me as an intelligent human being.

Now I grinned inwardly. I had told no one that I had a certain resistance to anaesthesia. After all, no one had asked. The anaesthetist glanced at me as he flipped the tourniquet off my arm and slowly, slowly, pushed the plunger into the syringe. I stared back in defiance, exhilarated to think that even now they could not put me down without a battle. Whilst my arm lay still and compliant, my spirit fought. I saw a slight flicker of anxiety cross the man's face as he glanced at my hard, challenging eyes and then at the level of drug left in the syringe. Finally, it began to usurp my consciousness, and I surrendered to the sensual creeping warmth and numbness; first legs and arms, then chest and neck until finally it reached, feather-like, into my face and throat. My eyes closed to the sound of rushing water in my head and a strange, swollen tingle on my lips. Was this what murderers experienced on execution? If so, it wasn't so bad.

A short time later I woke and spat out my airway. I lay quiet for a while trying to work out where I was and what had happened to me. Slowly memory returned and I felt my body and investigated my being to see how the convulsions had left me. A little tired, a slight headache, mainly hungry. I sat up.

Once the initial stimulus of a new experience had passed, I looked forward to electro-convulsive therapy only for the unorthodox anaesthetist and the sensual, painless sleep which his needle brought. ECT was administered to both the willing and the unwilling three mornings a week, so three mornings a week I went without breakfast and three mornings a week I lay with my head at the bottom of the bed while the cold conducting gel was placed on my temples. I was given a light general anaesthetic, then, once I was unconscious, electrodes were placed on the conducting gel, and some 70–120 volts of electricity were shot through my brain.

As time passed, like many ECT patients, I became haunted by fears that I would lose my memory. Sometimes when I came round, I couldn't remember who people were or where I was. It soon passed but what if one day it didn't? And what about the future? If still alive, what would my mind be like in twenty years' time?

On my return to the York Clinic, both Lily and Roland had vanished. They must have been out there somewhere, trying courageously to survive. How I missed my Roly! My dear protector, sage councillor, constant friend. How I longed for him to wrap his arms around me and hold me safe, rocking me, telling me not to be afraid. Now, more than ever, I felt I was fighting my battles alone.

Week after week they pumped electric shocks through my brains but, despite their hopes, I remained withdrawn, depressed, uncommunicative. After ten treatments had been extended to sixteen it was decided that the convulsions were not having the desired effect and so they moved on to a new cocktail of drugs.

7

Deep Sleep Treatment

LATER IT WAS generally agreed that an unusual drug combination had caused a toxic effect for, quite suddenly and otherwise inexplicably, I went truly mad—my mind foundered, or so I've been told. (Much of what follows I remember vividly, other parts have been threaded together from descriptions at the time.) Terror and anger were no longer guarded deep in the recesses of my soul; they were there in my hands as I tore off my clothes, in my legs and feet as I fled, frantic, from the ward. Anywhere. Away. I ran to the stairs and set off, panting, to the top of the building. Surely from there I could cast myself off and have done.

I found a door on the sixth floor and, all fear of doors forgotten, flung it open. Inside was a small room stacked high with clean linen. I clambered over the piles of sheets and towels and made for the skylight. It wouldn't open. With my fists I hammered at it in a frenzy to shatter the glass. Behind me, I could already hear footsteps on the stairs. I grabbed a chair and swung it with all my force against the glass. One leg of the chair splintered and hung down, impotent—but still the glass wouldn't break.

Hands seized me from behind and I fought them. No longer a quiet, passive Clare, I became a demon released at last, swinging the damaged chair at my assailants until they wrenched it from me. With arms flailing and bare feet kicking, I continued a powerful, mind-releasing orgy of aggression. Hurling abuse mingled with blows at the white-coated men, I was fighting for my freedom and integrity and would not be contained.

One of the men ran onto the landing and pressed an alarm. Reinforcements arrived. I was finally pinned down. Carried back to the ward, I arrived unkempt and utterly exhausted.

Sister Will appeared as, once released in my room, I again fought to be free.

"Now, Clare!" She was almost shouting, trying to penetrate my disintegration. She laid a firm hand on my arm and shook it, forcing me to pay attention. "Listen to me, Clare!" Again she shook me. "I want that you take this medicine."

In a flash my fist was out, knocking the plastic cup of sticky Largactil to the floor.[xx]

"I don't want any fucking medicine!" I shouted. "Bugger off! Leave me alone! Why the bloody hell can't you all get out of here and leave me alone!"

"Clare, you must control yourself. You will upset the other patients, and I am sure you don't want that."

I did. I wanted to set the whole stinking hospital on fire, punish it for my misery. I'd been good for so long, smothering myself in passivity. This madness was a liberating rampage. I wanted to be wild for ever. But through the exultant flames of fury, Sister's disapproval reawakened my lifelong enslavement to "being good", revived also my terror of causing harm. Finally, I buckled into silence.

"There now. That's better. What do you want that we do? Either you take the medicine, or we shall have to give you an injection. I don't want to do that, and I don't think you want it either."

With my brave, live anger burnt out, I was left with nothing but desolation and failure. I had tried to spread my wings and fly. They had come in force with a net and caught me and now they would clip those wings and put me back in my cage. Silently I accepted the new dose of medicine, then, climbing into bed, I buried my head under my pillow in bleak despair. It was the only privacy from prying eyes offered to the mentally sick. Sister Will gently stroked the sheets across my shoulders.

"That's right Clare. You have a good sleep." She pulled the curtains across the window and left me with a special nurse stationed once more at my door.

Next morning Dr Christie came in to see me.

"Well, I hear you've been airing your vocabulary for Sister. You must have been feeling pretty miserable, eh?" I lay, impassive as I had done ever since my abortive blast for freedom. I didn't care anymore, even for

Christie. If only I could stay in limbo, life must eventually die quietly of old age.

"Clare. Dr Fleminger and I feel this cannot go on. We have decided to give you a rest. Tomorrow morning, we are going to start a course of deep narcosis, sleep treatment you patients call it. How many ECTs have you had now?" I guess he asked the question merely to see if I would respond for, receiving no reply, he continued. "We've spoken to your parents, and they have given permission. They plan to go away for a well-earned holiday. Your troubles are a serious strain on them, you know."

I had wondered how long it would be before they punished me. *Let yourself go, they say. Let it all hang out. Show us how you feel. And when you do they mash your brains with electricity or fill your veins with drugs or put you to sleep like a rabid dog. And why do they always say they have my parents' permission? Is it to make me feel it's all right? That 'Mummy' and 'Daddy' say so. Or is it to rub in my powerlessness?*[xxi]

"Okay. Well..." He rose awkwardly to his feet, perhaps pondering how it was that I managed to make him feel as if he was persecuting me instead of trying his level best to stop me from throwing my life away. "I'll pop in and see you settled down tomorrow morning and then you can have a long sleep and forget your troubles for a while."

Forget? How much more do they want me to forget? Without memories how will I know who I am, what I stand for, what moral code I believe in? They could wipe me out, transform me into whatever they please. I told no one of my fears, not even David, for my recent experiences had cut me off from the outside world; I had travelled beyond Dave's power of imagining.

The following day I bathed, put on a clean hospital gown, was given two suppositories and escorted to the lavatory. I didn't mind. I had long since relinquished custody of my body, fighting only to retain custody of my mind.

On returning to my room, I found it transformed. The high bed frame had been wheeled out into the corridor and on the floor, in its place, was a mattress laid on a plastic sheet. A faint flame of interest flickered then died. There was no longer enough life in me to kindle it. The yellow curtains were pulled against the morning sun leaving the room washed by a yellowish tinge.

"There we are, Clare, now you take these tablets and then into bed and have a good rest." Sister, while smiling at me, spoke to me as if to an infant. They didn't seem to realise that I was past caring what they did to me. They had already slowed my mind with their shocks and now they were taking even consciousness away.

Obediently I swallowed the drugs and sank onto the mattress on the floor. *Well, chum, you can't get any lower than this if you try!*

A nurse pulled a chair close to the top of the mattress, just out of my field of vision, and sat down.

"And so the prisoner rests," I murmured.

"What?"

"Doesn't matter."

For twenty-two hours out of twenty-four over the next month I slept. When I emerged from sleep every four or five hours, I was unaware of my surroundings. But assuming they followed the procedures laid down in old nursing manuals, the nurses would have washed me, spoon-fed me sloppy food, taken me to the lavatory, brushed my hair, cleaned my teeth, massaged my pressure areas, powdered me, straightened the sheets and then given me more drugs. They would have kept frequent checks on my pulse and blood pressure. No doubt a doctor came each day to oscillate my chest for signs of congestion, incipient pneumonia. It is difficult and time-consuming nursing patients in deep narcosis: indeed it had led to a number of deaths, but it also provides a rare experience for medical and nursing students. In my case, at the time, I thought they undertook it in the hope that, as I became more and more drugged, I would forget my past intransigence and be more amenable to new ways of thinking. I guessed the idea was to change my thought processes. But maybe it was deeper than that. Maybe they had realised I had some remorseless memory buried deep inside me, a memory that needed to be expunged before I went quite mad.

* * *

When I woke four weeks later, there was a nurse still sitting on a chair.

"Hello, Clare. How do you feel?"

I looked slowly round. I drew the words out through my drug-drenched brain. They echoed distantly but held no meaning. *How do I feel? How do you feel? How should I feel? Why should I feel? I. Who am I? I? I? Clare. Clare who? Who is Clare? Clare is me? Clare who? I'm sure I had another name. What was it? Clare what?* My chest constricted in panic. I couldn't even remember my name!

Laboriously I tried to piece together the objects around me, to fit them into a coherent whole. *Why am I lying on the floor? Why do people lie on the floor and what is making the air yellow? It's all yellow. The world is yellow. It never was—at least, I don't think it was...?*

The narcosis had catalysed grotesquely with the convulsions and drugs in my brain to produce a quagmire of confusion.

A man walked into the room. My short-sighted eyes saw his shoes advancing towards me. I knew they were men's shoes, but how did I know? The man bent down. He was good looking with thick dark hair and slightly protruding brown eyes. He seemed to know me. How did I know he knew me? Why *did* he know me?

"Ah! Good. You've woken up, Clare. You've been asleep for a long time, now we must get you up and about." He paused. "Tomorrow we'll move your bed back in here and then you'll feel more yourself."

I heard him but I couldn't understand what he was saying. He stopped and spoke more slowly. "Do you understand me, Clare? You've had a long sleep. Now you can wake up." He was raising his voice as if I was a foreign tourist. He felt my pulse, looked at my pupils. "Right. Well, I'll go along now and let you sleep some more. I'll look in again later."

I lay still for a while trying to grasp what he had said. He said I had been asleep but why couldn't I remember anything? I turned to the nurse.

"Who is he?" I found it hard to modulate my voice, it was so long since last I spoke.

"Why, Dr Christie of course!" Her voice was full of surprise.

"But who *is* he?" I hated to ask but I had to know. Despite remembering almost nothing, despite those hundreds of hours of deep sleep, I knew I was hugely vulnerable and that *they* were my enemies, *they* were trying to break into my core, to reveal my iniquity. Now it was vital that I remember who *they* were.

"He's your doctor," the nurse said. And then, more gently, "Don't you remember him?" She looked down at me with pity, where I lay on the floor. She was just about my age and there I was, flat on my back with no more hope left in me, being nursed like a baby and now I appeared to have lost my memory as well.

"No. No I don't remember him at all." My voice trailed away.

He said I've been asleep for a long time. Why? Am I ill? Have I had an operation? What if they've cut off my legs or breasts or severed my brain? I sat up and, as if drunk, folded back the bed clothes with exaggerated deliberation. The nurse watched me anxiously.

"Do you want a bed pan?"

I looked up, my eyes out of focus. The words meant nothing at all, and I returned to my silent exploration. I vaguely saw two legs, grown thin from inaction. Gingerly I felt my body under the hospital gown. Nothing seemed cut or sore or bruised. So why was I lying on the floor and why was a strange doctor visiting me? Gradually the drugs reclaimed me, and I drifted once more into sleep.

* * *

The process of recreating my past was so all consuming, so emotionally draining that my previous defiance diminished. Gradually, day by day, I surrendered little bits of the Clare Thompson that I was discovering for Christie's scrutiny. Up till then my therapy sessions had been dominated by the fear that if I told him anything at all of my past, relinquished even the thinnest layer of my defences, he would have the key to my destruction. Then their treatment had blasted my past into splintered atoms, a thousand dead slivers of knowledge.

One day I was sitting in Christie's consulting room.

"Did I ever tell you I had a little brother?"

"No!" Christie sounded surprised.

"He was called Richard. I've been thinking a lot about him lately. I don't know why. No one really talks about him anymore. I loved him. I still remember his birthday. December 6th."

"What happened?"

I looked down at the 'sanity table'. "I have some really vivid memories of him. At least I think I do. But maybe it's just things I've put together. I can't tell any more. I must have been about three. I see him sitting on my mother's lap. Lots of black hair and a big head. I remember a low-ceilinged bedroom with oak beams. My mother trying to feed him raw eggs. He was sick. He cried. It was not long after the war. Eggs were rationed, precious. If he refused to eat them then I had to. And I hated them. Slimy. I'd refuse and make a big fuss."

"How long was he sick?"

"I don't know. I don't think I ever asked. Maybe half a year. Maybe more. He got meningitis. You know, it infected the membrane round his brain. They treated him with sulphanilamide, one of the very earliest antibiotics, shipped in specially for him from the States. But it was too late. Eventually they tried to operate on him, to drain the liquid inside his brain. But he died on the operating table. My uncle was the anaesthetist. He said Richard would have been blind and deaf if he'd survived. But I loved him. When he died my mother went away for a while. Was it my fault that she'd gone away? Was it because of me making all that fuss? Is that why she left? Was that why Richard disappeared too, for it must have felt like that to a three-year-old. Was it because I'd been bad? Then this cold woman, my mother's stepmother, who had no children and who I sensed instinctively disliked them, came to look after us instead. When my mother came back, she let me have Richard's favourite cuddly toy. It was a little blue and grey plush figure of Piglet, only Richard had loved him so much all the plush had worn off. Piglet was so small I could get my thumb and index finger right round his neck. I took him to bed with me every night for years. A little bit of Richard."

As each piece of memory was surrendered to the psychiatrists, I disowned it as if it was no longer a part of me. Thus, slowly, I approached the true centre of my terror, that all-powerful source of malevolence which now grew daily within me, and which I truly believed, if revealed, would unleash upon the world an essence of malignancy of such magnitude that all would be destroyed. But I didn't know what it was. I just knew that I harboured it inside me. Even in my exhaustion this black essence had to be guarded with constant vigilance against all intruders. Beside it, all the periphery became insignificant.

I no longer remember how long I lay there nor at what point it was decided there was no more they could do for me, that it was time for me to go home.

8

Home

LYING ALONE UNDER my favourite oak tree, I gazed bleakly up into its branches. The leaves had grown darker with the heightening sun while the grass on the lawn yellowed in one of the hottest summers in living memory.[xxii] But that year, inside my parents' pebbledash-clad house, summer never came. Instead, I had come home. I had dreaded this return when my guilt would confront me daily in my mother's greying hair and gaunt face. Was it guilt, too, that made me feel so bitter? Made me bolt from the house to walk endlessly through the nearby woods, brooding? Only last night I had felt nauseous and had turned down the chicken Mum had cooked. She had tried to persuade me to eat it, becoming somewhat overbearing in her anxiety, and I'd sworn and flung from the table, my insides knotted with self-reproach and anger and hopelessness. Sometimes I wanted to shout at them, these kind, much-loved parents of mine, "I'm alive, aren't I? That's what you want isn't it? You can't expect me to be nice as well. God damn it, I never asked to be born!"

I probably loved my mother more than anyone in the world and yet now I avoided her, hiding away in my room or out in the garden, as the blackness inside me worked its outward destruction. My homecoming had turned life into a burden for her. I had become a curse. She had lost weight, grown older through months of living on edge, no doubt searching for some explanation, some answer to the single question: why? A question I myself couldn't answer. The pain, yes, that was obvious. But why this terrible inner darkness? I looked at my watch, an action which had recently begun to fill me with strange disquiet. It was tea-time.

I could imagine them now, drinking tea companionably together in the old playroom furnished with a magnificent, Regency, mahogany, glass-doored bookcase that my father, a great lover of antiques and haunter of auction houses, had snapped up for a song. Against one wall stood my mother's upright piano, now seldom heard. They would no doubt be sitting in the comfy, worn armchairs trying, yet again, to make sense of the whole ruddy mess.

Did Dad bring out his old adage on parenting? "The parents' job is to create a loving home, to set a good example of kindness and honesty—and then to stand back and be ready to catch the children if they fall." Right now, they were catching me.

Pa[xxiii] was such a dear, wise man. Not always very good at communicating with his children, especially me and Dave, but we're all made differently. Sometimes Mum must have wished that he had been more forceful, hadn't left all the disciplining to her, but then that was his nature: kind, retiring and with a lovely, gentle sense of humour. At least at home. What, I used to wonder, was he like in charge of his troops? He couldn't have risen to being a brigadier general without leadership qualities. He had taught all of us that the place to lead from was the front—and if you had a problem, always take it to the top to find a solution.

I got slowly to my feet, rubbed my arms where the harsh, dry grass stalks had left red welts on my skin. I should go in and see if Mum needed help. Food still had to be cooked, and dishes washed despite the present turmoil. I went back inside to the large, old-fashioned kitchen, where Mum had dumped their tea tray by the sink alongside the dirty plates left over from lunch. I started to wash up, watching as she cleared a space on the well-scrubbed wooden table.

"I'm doing steak and kidney pie for supper, one of your father's favourites," she called out. "I hope you'll eat it."

"Of course," I replied, trying to keep the edge out of my voice. Mum had probably realised that, lately, she had spent too much time worrying about me and not enough in comforting her husband.

Crossing the kitchen she went into the larder, a room icy cold in winter but pleasantly cool in even the most sweltering summer. From a marble shelf she took the butter and then went to the store cupboard to collect the flour and salt for the pie crust. Making pastry soothed her nerves.

Washing up. It had been a bone of contention when we all came home from boarding school for the holidays. That is, until Mum drew up a strict rota. John then wrote a poem and stuck it above the old stone sink in the scullery:

When you do the washing-up
Of breakfast, dinner, tea or sup,
Please be sure to do the lot,
Every filthy pan and pot!

My thoughts drifted back to those early days when we had first moved to High Beech, and to my older brother, John. As a child, six years his junior, I'd half worshipped him but, intermittently, I'd hated him as well. He could be so bossy, trying to rule not only Dave and me but our parents too. David had learnt to avoid head-on confrontations. Except once.

I must have been around seven. Together, we children had built a den out of bits of wood and plywood at the foot of another of the old trees in our unkempt garden. John had spent much of the morning provoking Dave. Slowly the tension had risen until, suddenly, John announced that the den was his and tried to push David out.

Dave, reaching explosion point, caught John unawares, managed to knock him from squatting near the entry to lying flat on his back on the ground. Scrambling astride him, Dave then grabbed John's ears and began hammering his head against the hard-packed earth shouting in frenzy, "I'm going to kill you! I'm going to kill you!"

Terrified, I believed every word and ran for help. The first person I found was Mum. Together we went to my father. Told that his younger son was trying to murder his older one, he had looked up abstractedly from the typewriter where he was banging out an article.

'Oh dear, love, what should we do?' With that, Mum became furious. Furious at her husband's lack of forcefulness and at her children for their bickering. Small as she was, she stomped off to the den, grabbed Dave by the scruff of his neck and, shouting, "Stop it at *once!*" dragged him to his feet and sent him to his room. Then she turned on John. "As for you, I've no doubt you started it. You stay right here until I send for you!" And she marched into the house and disappeared.

None of us had ever seen Mum so angry, ever heard her shout at us, or use physical force against us. It was a moment we wouldn't forget. And I, the watching, frightened child, had wanted first to comfort John.

Our wandering existence provided few certainties. Now even Mum's self-control, Dave's gentleness, and, most of all, John's dominance had all been shattered. John, the all-powerful, the idol, had been reduced to the tears he so proudly scorned. His image smashed, I wanted fervently to rebuild it. But surely John would box my ears if I offered him comfort, so I crept away to the attic to console my long-time ally, Dave. He who protected me and talked to me and was my friend. Yet, in that moment of unforgivable disloyalty, I had been willing to sacrifice him for the sake of repairing my fallen god.

An hour or so later I remembered Mum. She, too, had been frighteningly upset. Where had she gone? I hunted through every room of the Edwardian, eight-bedroomed house. Over and over, I called out, "Mummy! Mummy!" It was growing dark outside but still I couldn't find her.

I went to my father. "Daddy, where's Mummy?"

"I don't know Poppet. She must be around somewhere."

"She's *not!*" I screamed and ran downstairs. I was convinced that my mother had left. My parents almost never quarrelled, so, to me, this row seemed catastrophic.

I finally ended up huddled on the floor in a corner of the cold scullery by the back door, waiting and waiting for my mother to return. Once I ventured out into the garden but there in the dark, the tall hedges and trees became dreadful things of fear sheltering I knew not what. I returned indoors to my silent vigil.

Who knows how long I sat there, but at last I heard footsteps. I pulled open the back door, ran up the path and flung myself, sobbing, into my mother's arms.

"I thought you'd left us, Mummy! I looked everywhere! I thought you'd never come back. Oh Mummy, don't leave us. Please don't!"

My mother held me close and said, half-apologetically, "I didn't think anyone would notice I'd gone. I needed a walk." I clung more tightly to her then, just to make sure she knew I loved her.

It was now three months since the deep narcosis. The restoration of my wall of memories was pretty much as good as it was going to get. Considerable gaps still remained—and do to this day—and my previous mental agility was apparently lost for ever. I sensed another upsurge of depression rolling towards me. It seemed to come now in regular waves, when all my self-hatred, my sense of evil, of fear, rose in front of me, a cresting breaker of overpowering force; when the unknown terror rushed at me and I saw a green river flowing from me, pervading the corners of the earth and I knew I was dutybound to destroy myself, to save the world from my iniquity.

For several days the conflict had been raging. One moment a voice would tell me to think of my parents and what my death would do to them. But then that other self counter-attacked. *But look what you've done to them already. Alive you're destroying them. You cloud Mum's life with your darkness. If only you were dead, she could live free, free from the shame and fear of you, her daughter. Look in her eyes, secretly searching your face to check if she's doing the right thing. You're destroying her. But it is you that must be destroyed.*

Getting up, I walked silently up to my room. It was time to do my duty.

As night and sleep enfolded the stone house, I made my final preparations. I signed a couple of cheques to clear my debts and tucked them under a book on my bedside table. Then I wrote out my favourite Shakespeare sonnet:

No longer mourn for me when I am dead,
Than you shall hear the surly sullen bell
Give warning to the world that I am fled,
From this vile world with vilest worms to dwell.
Nay if you read this line, remember not
The hand that writ it; for I love you so,

That I in your sweet thoughts would be forgot,
If thinking on me then should make you woe.
O if I say, you look upon this verse
When I perhaps compounded am with clay,
Do not so much as my poor name rehearse,
But let your love even with my life decay;
Lest the wise world should look into your moan,
And mock you with me after I am gone.

This I folded in half and placed into an envelope addressed to my parents. Then, quite calmly, I felt for my pulse and, with a fresh razor blade, cut down in search of the artery. I couldn't find it! To this day I don't know why. I tried five times, twice on my right wrist and three times on the left but only an ooze of blood escaped, not the fountain I was hunting for. So I slipped into my faithful blue dressing gown and, carrying my eiderdown, I stole downstairs to the gas stove in the back kitchen. It was time for Plan B. I turned on the gas and, wrapping the eiderdown around me to block out any air, I put my head in the oven.

As I smelt the gas a momentary fear seized me, a memory of my first operation as a small child: a gas mask clamped to my face, suffocating and struggling to get free while the giant hand held firm. Giant hands. They were killing me. He was killing me. I could not escape. I was helpless. Hands trying to destroy me. Then I calmed myself. This was, after all, quite different. I was in control. I could always pull my head out if I wanted to. But I had made a pact with the world. I had sworn I would rid it of my malevolence and that pact must not be broken.

Unconsciousness seemed a long time coming.

Much later my father told me his side of the story. In their king-sized bed, my parents slept side by side. As always since my return, they kept their bedroom door slightly ajar, their senses never totally relaxed. Dad lay beside Mum in exhausted, uneasy sleep. He was trying to write a book. A deadline loomed. But he found it hard to concentrate. Affairs at home obtruded into his thoughts more than probably most people realised. He worried about both his beloved Ro and me.

It had been hard to find himself, even at a distance, in collusion with the psychiatrists, but he was confused and unsure and, in his bewilderment, turned to the doctors, the experts with experience of such things, and tried to co-operate. At least the York Clinic was well known. With me home, the added responsibility weighed on him although my presence in the outside world, like the first lambing of spring, was surely a sign for hope. But what was my visit doing to poor Ro? Should he perhaps find a flat for me before I drove his adored wife to her own nervous breakdown? I seemed so bitter and hostile, so unpredictable now. He told me later that it was nerve-wracking picking his way round my problems so as to maintain a semblance of peace. Mental illness seemed as dangerous and communicable as cholera.

That night he stirred in his sleep and his brain surfaced momentarily into conscious thought as he heard my door across the landing quietly open and a floorboard creek. He knew he should investigate but he was too wrapped in sleep to do more than register the sound before plunging once more into his dreams.

* * *

The casualty officer sewed up my wrists without resource to local anaesthetic. Then the oxygen mask was removed, leaving me gasping for air, dragging me back into consciousness. I was still alive. As the doctor tugged the needle through my resisting flesh for the last time, the kitchen gas reclaimed me, and I slept.

Next morning a tall, angular man advanced down the women's ward of the local hospital. Instantly I knew he was a psychiatrist and I his prey. I turned my head away, dreading the never-ending round of psychiatrists and institutions striding into my life again. For a moment the man stood over me without speaking. I kept my head still, my eyes level with his belt buckle.

"Miss Thompson?" His voice sounded a little detached but not cold. Slowly, wearily, I rolled my head back on the pillow to look at him. I wanted so much to hibernate forever in some dark fissure in the earth, far from modern psychiatric treatment. I should have jumped from a bridge. It could not be more painful than the ministrations of these mental can openers.

"I'm Dr Stead.[xxiv] Sister has asked me to have a word with you. Perhaps we could go to her office."

I considered the possibility of playing dead, of simply ignoring him. But inevitably, it would be noted in my file and might later lead to some further 'treatment'. I had had enough treatment. I had indeed learnt my lesson. I would conform.

I sat up without enthusiasm and, while the doctor hovered, I slipped my feet into a new pair of fluffy slippers, bought for me by my mother to celebrate my return home. Doing up the buttons on my dressing gown hurt my stitched and bandaged wrists so I gave up and, trying to hide myself inside its worn, familiar folds, I followed him down the ward to Sister's office, glancing at the other patients. Had they, too, recognised this man as a psychiatrist and myself, *ipso facto*, as insane?

"Do have a seat, Miss Thompson." I noticed at once that the office had no sanity table, for the room was usually used only by the staff, the *ipso facto* sane. "Miss Thompson, I've been asked to visit you to see if perhaps I can help you." He said it half as a question, leaving me to answer or not as I wished. I was soon to learn that Dr Stead had built up a practice, and reputation, by concentrating his work on younger patients who had failed to respond to other psychiatrists' therapies. Unknown to me, I was being considered as a possible candidate for an elite band of the mentally sick. I did not stir or look up.

"I gather you were seeing Dr Christie at the York Clinic."

"Yes." I cleared my throat and continued to avoid his eyes.

"He has left the Clinic now you know but he says he will see you if you wish."

Dr Christie? I had grown very fond of him, perhaps too fond, for some deep, underlying instinct for health told me that he could never uncover and exorcise my ghosts and make me well.

On the other hand, Dr Stead was an unknown quantity—and posed one serious threat. I was now not in London but near my hometown,

Haywards Heath, that place dominated by St Francis' 19th century, 800 bed, lunatic asylum, a vast building, apparently a mating between a Victorian laundry and a prison, its grounds surrounded by high walls.[xxv]

"I won't go to St Francis!"

Dr Stead appeared startled by my sudden vehemence.

"You don't want to go to St Francis?" Too late I realised I had offered him a glimpse of emotion, a crack in my armour which he could one day use against me.

"No. I *won't* go." I spat out the words. Dr Stead waited a moment, giving me time to explain myself. When no explanation was forthcoming, he carried on smoothly.

"As a matter of fact, I'm in charge of a small hospital on the south coast, the Lady Chichester Hospital, where we thought you might stay for a while as you get better. I think you'd like it." Now he lent towards me, his body taut in his earnestness. "I'm willing to try and help you, Miss Thompson, but I can only take you on if you are willing to work with me."

I kept my face impassive. But I was sifting anxiously through the signals the man was sending out. *'We thought,' so, once more, I really have no say in the matter. 'I'm willing to try and help you but...' If I accept, I have to pledge allegiance to his side.*

I wondered what the alternatives were. If I refused, would they take me by force and incarcerate me in St Francis? What if I asked to go home? Asked my parents to save me? But that would be cruel in a way that trying to kill myself had not been. Then I had been attempting to save them from me. Begging them to save me from the psychiatrists would throw them into a conflict between what the experts prescribed and what I, their daughter, demanded. And what if they chose the psychiatrists? What if I lost the vote?

Eventually I agreed as ungraciously as I could, attempting to minimise any commitment to co-operate.

"Good! I think we should work well together."

Dr Stead stood up and shook my hand. I was to discover that the doctor's old-world courtesy, extending as it did even to his patients, inspired great loyalty among them. With a wistful smile on his rather gaunt face he said,

"Goodbye."

As he went in search of the ward sister to arrange my transfer, I wondered why he lumbered himself with people like me. Clearly failure carried less onus if someone else had failed first. Later I was to get to know some of his other patients. Nearly all were young, intelligent, with many years of health ahead of them—if only he could find the key to unlock it. He was a last port of call in the storm. If he, too, gave up on us, we would end up on some closed ward of St Francis, totally shut off from the living world.

I walked back past the long line of beds, feeling unutterably alone. They would all say that it was for my own good, that I was to be stripped of my most buried memories. My black terror and shame ripped open and laid bare. And there was no one on earth to defend me. Recently it had inched into my consciousness that my world had, quite literally, turned grey. Even the flowers and birds had lost their colour, to match the grey inside me.

I climbed into bed and buried my head under the pillow, engulfed within its blackness, hiding from prying eyes. I set up a gentle rocking motion to ease the pain in my arm and to comfort my lonely heart.

The ward lights were out, everyone else asleep, but I continued rocking deep into the night. The pink draught of chloral hydrate did nothing to calm my brain or ease the pain. Then, from far away, I felt a hand placed softly on my shoulder and I crouched still, fear pulsing in my throat. Gently the night doctor on call, lifted the pillow from my head and sat close to me on the bed.

Moonlight streamed through a large window and lit up his face. I blinked and looked again. He was profoundly disfigured, his face raw and puckered from terrible burns. I, too, was disfigured—but on the inside where only I could see it. A pain shot up my arm, jerked through my body and registered itself in a contraction of my face. He felt the jolt.

"What's the matter, Clare? Can you tell me?" His voice was deep with the desire to understand.

"It's nothing. Just the pain in my arm."

"Have you had it long?"

"Six years."

"That's long."

"No one seems able to cure it. They operated. Found the nerve wrapped around my first rib. They cut the rib out. But it did nothing for the pain. In fact, it made it worse. And so then they implied it was my fault. All in my mind. But it isn't. It's not in my head. It's in my arm!"

"What do you take for it?"

"Nothing. They don't prescribe painkillers for psychological pain."

"Would you like me to write you up for something?"

I looked at him with incredulity. I stammered in my disbelief. "W-would you? Would you really? It would make *such* a difference! No one seems to realise how demoralising chronic pain is. If I could just stop the pain perhaps..." my voice trailed off into the moonlight, leaving the hope hanging in the air between us.

"Perhaps I know a little how you feel. I've had quite a bit of pain myself. Hang on and I'll get you something."

The night doctor rose silently from the bed to fetch the drugs and returned a few minutes later with two DF118. I swallowed them gratefully.

In less than an hour the pills had worked. It was unbelievable. I was FREE FROM PAIN! I kept checking to make sure. All those years and just two little pills and it had gone. Why had no one ever bothered to try that before? Because I was a girl—so my pain must be psychological? Pain so unrelenting that I tried to kill myself, my life not worth living, and not one soul had offered me strong analgesics—until now.[xxvi]

I had said that if only the pain went, I would be able to walk out into the world, get a job, find a flat. Now bleak certainty told me I couldn't. Not anymore. I was no longer fit to face the world. With their drugs and their shocks and their deep narcosis, they had changed me. I had also changed myself with that haunting darkness skulking inside me. Most of all, though, by implying over and over again that I was damaged, mentally unsound, they had crushed my self-belief.

A Red Cross driver came to transport me to Dr Stead's 'hospital by the sea'. Summer had passed its zenith and rain had put new life into the tired trees. The orchards' red fruits gleamed like ripe baubles. Momentarily, I felt at peace.

9

The Lady Chichester

THE LADY CHICHESTER Hospital, housed in a detached Edwardian building set in its own grounds, stood a short walk from the sea.[xxvii] During the day the front door was always unlocked so most of the patients could come and go as they pleased. Inside, the white paint on the walls had turned dingy, the wooden floors were bare, the windows lacked curtains. It was a poor man's loony bin, a provincial funny farm.

But it was not only the building that was different. The York Clinic had been attached to a world-class teaching hospital and drew most of its staff from the cream of the country's psychiatric professionals. At the Lady Chich, as the patients affectionately called it, several of the nursing and junior medical staff seemed, at least to me, slightly more unbalanced than the patients they were paid to serve—and considerably less astute.

At the York Clinic most of the patients, apart from Lily, were on their best behaviour. Only under extreme stress did they conduct themselves in anything other than a civilized, middle-class manner. To them a spade was a horticultural implement. At the Chich a spade was a spade; frequently used for digging shit. Here, for the first time, I heard the word 'lunatic' used by a patient in reference to herself. It came without connotations of shame; rather it carried a slight sense of devil-may-care pride with a touch of bitter cynicism. These patients ridiculed themselves to pre-empt other's derision. 'Loony bin' was a phrase we used frequently. We had earned the right to skip the euphemisms.

Lady Chichester patients accepted that they were outcasts, misfits. But surrounded by a staff who, frequently, were separated from them only by a technicality of diagnosis and uniform, the patients developed a strong possessiveness towards the hospital; it was theirs, an island of neurosis and psychosis, a haven for nutcases and loonies. The Chich engendered a strange loyalty verging on fondness.

In this enclosed world, Dr Stead's cases formed the upper echelons. Just by virtue of being under him, I found I had been accorded a place amongst the elite, while my large number of treatments put me near the pinnacle of that upside-down world where dominance and respect depended on how many treatments/psychiatrists had been resisted, how many barbiturates were needed to produce sleep, how much Largactil needed to produce calm, and how many 'years sick' a person was.

Here, I discovered others who shared my fear that if they were totally known, understood, they would be annihilated. I realized, sardonically, that here, at last, I belonged. No Stead patient ever reassured another by saying, "You'll soon be better!" For each of them harboured a hidden dread that 'better' would mean capitulation.

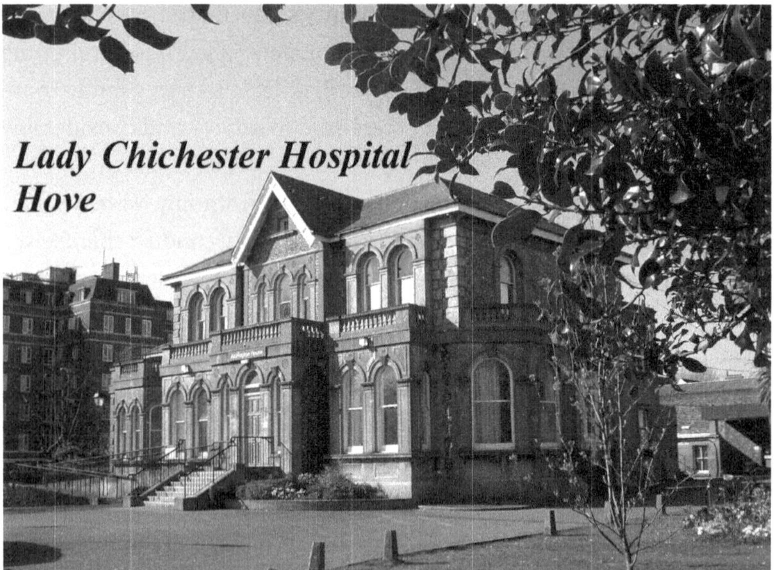

The Lady Chichester. [Credit: Joe Hughes]

The main, all-women's building boasted several wards. The long, dark admissions, or Alexandra Ward and general ward were on the first floor, with an annex on one side for those who had been there for some weeks and had been granted the freedom of street clothes. Out on the other side was Ann Ward, or the 'sunroom', with skylights and windows looking down to the sea. This room housed long-term patients, mainly alcoholics and drug addicts, who had yet to graduate to street clothing. A few doors up the road, terraced buildings housed the men's and the children's annex.

On arrival, my street clothes were labelled and taken away. The contents of my sponge bag were examined. I was given a bath to which disinfectant had been added. In under an hour I had been stripped of my identity, depersonalized; even my germs had been taken away. I was then showed into the ten-patient ward, led to an empty bed one from the end on the left-hand side and told to stay there until the resident doctor came to see me.

Near midnight on my second day, Dr Hallow finally arrived, a pasty-faced woman with an overweight waddle. I had been warned about her.

"Wait till you see Dr Hallow! She's really screwed up." Pauline, a woman in her thirties, had spoken with a touch of loathing in her voice.

"Screwed being the operative word. I better warn you, she has a particular fondness for teenage girls." And Hannah, a quiet girl with beautiful, high Slavic cheek bones, gave a disdainful, half-ironic smile.

"She'll come for you in the middle of the night." Pauline went on. "They say she's scared of the dark so makes us keep her company. Just make sure you keep your knickers on."

"I wouldn't mind so much," chipped in Carol, a middle-aged grandmother, "if she'd only come before they'd given out the night sedation. You can never get back to sleep after."

"And she's scared of microbes. She gets the children in the annex to scrub the corridors with disinfectant every day. I promise you. She's got raw rims of flesh round her wrists!" Hannah's eyes were now twinkling, like a mischievous child telling horror stories after dark.

Dr Hallow's sickness had reached mythical proportions. And while patients were usually exceptionally sensitive to the fears of their comrades, they could be quite vicious if similar weaknesses were found on the other side of the sanity table.

That night Dr Hallow led me to her small consulting room, closed the door and, as she vigorously scrubbed her hands and arms, told me to undress. Remembering Pauline's advice, I kept my knickers firmly in place. Then I stood stock still, braced and scared. I could no longer bear the thought of being touched; of someone else taking possession of my body. And yet I mustn't let this woman know. For, deep down in my subconscious, I knew that my fear of being touched was part of my malaise.

The doctor's eyes scanned my body from head to toe, before returning to linger around my breasts. Then she advanced towards me and, putting one arm firmly around my shoulders, with the other hand she examined, massaged, each breast inch by inch. My body trembled and I flushed deep red with disgust at myself as I saw my nipples involuntarily harden and stand proud.

"Right. Take your knickers off and climb up on the table." For a second I looked at the woman in misery. Then I quickly closed my eyes to hide my fear. What could I do? What if I ran from the room? Would it not all be distorted and interpreted in those grisly files? Would not Dr Stead get to hear of my "intransigence"?

I did as I was told.

The doctor leant over the table, stroking her hands down either side of my long, slim body, feeling again my ripe breasts as they lay, flaccid now, defeated. Then Dr Hallow moved her hands towards my stomach. I could not help myself. I let out an involuntary cry, clasped my navel and curled my knees up in defence.

"Oh please don't!" I whispered. "I'm ticklish!" *God! No one, but no one must touch me there.* The very thought made my want to retch. The doctor paused, a slight twist to her lips, and then went to a side table. She took a rubber glove from the kidney dish and lubricated her index and middle fingers with KY Jelly.

"Right, put your knees up. I'm going to give you an internal. Come on. Legs apart!" The woman parted my legs and then my pubic hair, before forcing her two fingers hard inside my vagina. There she twisted and turned her hand until sweat appeared on her pallid forehead and upper lip. I fled, eyes closed, in search of that other place, that limbo where nothing and nobody could reach me.

"Okay. On your side. Let's check the other end." And the woman violated me again. Finally, she finished. As she stripped off the glove and returned to the sink, she told me to sit on the chair by the desk. Still dazed with shock, I slipped my nightdress over my head and then put on my knickers. The woman should be sacked. But if I complained, would they not say I had imagined it? That I was sexually frustrated, or deviant, and was making the whole thing up? Might they not start at last to peer into my sexual being, the place where I was, for some strange reason, more than anywhere else, petrified that they might enter. She finally released me at two in the morning.

On my return to the ward all was in darkness except where the moon cast shafts of light across the well-worn floorboards. In the bed next to mine Hannah lay, eyes wide open, watching.

"How was it?" Hannah's voice was gentle, full of sympathy.

My body began once more to shake. My voice quavered as I whispered back, "Horrible! Absolutely horrible! Why can't we do something? The woman's sick. We ought to report her."

"You can't. Someone tried. The staff refused to believe them. She was a patient, right? Obviously deluded. But you should be alright now. Con never pursues anyone who doesn't invite pursuit."

"But what about the children? She sleeps over there with them."

Hannah lay still. Later she was to tell me about her own childhood. How she had had to sleep with her father in his bed until suddenly, one day, he had kicked her out, turned against her, had chosen her younger sister instead and barely spoke to Hannah again. She, too, had wondered about the children.

* * *

It was not until the fourth day that I was summoned to see Dr Stead. An elderly nurse escorted me downstairs.

"Dr Stead's room's being redecorated so he's seeing you in there. That's the day room." The nurse pointed at a closed door and left.

A sweat broke out down my back. *Why are doors always closed against me?* I shut my eyes, clenched my fists and forced myself to knock. Then I opened the door as if it were the gateway to Hades.

"Ah, Miss Thompson! Come on in." Dr Stead had risen to his feet and held out his hand, invariably courteous and respectful to his patients. "Have a seat."

The room was large, light and airy, furnished with a remarkable assortment of chairs. I approached them with alarm. Months of living under psychiatric scrutiny had made me wary of anything unusual. Were these chairs a deliberate trap, like the coloured triangles, to measure my difference? For once I regretted that there was no sanity table to tell me where to sit. If I sat on the deep sofa, would I be hiding myself away or, if I chose the stool, was that infantile or too humble? The hard, straight chairs no doubt showed masochistic tendencies. It never occurred to my troubled mind that the chairs were merely a hotchpotch of what was available for group therapy sessions. It is thus that psychiatric hospitals create psychiatric patients. I chose a pouf, hoping it showed a blend of the comfortable and the not too low, modern and yet not too far from him to look afraid.

"Sorry about the mess but they're redecorating my office." He smiled but his eyes were calculating, not hard so much as astute. Despite the fact that, thanks to the DF118, my pain was almost gone, I sat as usual with my arm clutched to my stomach, my legs crossed, my back arched forward a little. I waited, gently rocking to ease the tension.

Dr Stead watched me for a moment and then said in a quiet, even voice, "Why are you so afraid Miss Thompson? Are you scared we will discover something you want to hide from us, from everyone?"

The words hit with crushing clarity. He knew. He understood. In one sentence he had pierced to my core fear, that someone one day would break in and reveal something vile. The question hung heavy in the air between us. What should I say?

Ever since losing my memory, doubts and fears of insanity had closed in until I was now almost convinced I was mad. This man would know. He would not let me tie him in knots with pretended sanity. Or was it insanity that I was faking? I no longer knew but maybe he could save me. He could also annihilate me.

I watched intently as he rearranged his legs. Absently I started to pick at fluff on my dressing gown, keeping my eyes down so that he could not see inside my mind. Our silence lengthened oppressively. *What am I supposed to say? What does he want me to do?*

"Are you feeling nervous, Miss Thompson?" I stopped plucking at my dressing gown and clasped my hands around my knees instead.

"A little." I tried to be noncommittal but instead managed to sound sulky.

"Do you want to tell me about it?" His voice was quiet and controlled, his pose still, like a chameleon awaiting its prey.

I shrugged my shoulders in their tired blue robe and again the silence grew bloated between us.

"I don't know what you want me to say."

He laughed softly in genuine amusement. "You're not giving much away, are you?" In an instant he was serious. He leant forward, his legs untwined, no longer relaxed. The trouble with difficult patients was to get them started; that was, after all, why they were difficult. "You're sick Miss Thompson, we all know that. I think we can help to make you well again, but not if you fight us. We've got to work together to discover what it is that has made you so afraid. Then I think we can beat it. But I can't work with you if I don't know how you feel. You must help." He spoke with the earnest naivety of a schoolboy. Did he really believe they could make me unafraid?

"I feel I have to kill myself. It's my obligation." I flung it out as a challenge, or was it a threat? Was I trying to tell him I would rather die than get 'better', than find out why I was so afraid?

"What makes you feel that?"

"Has no one told you? Surely in that great dossier on my every movement there must be some revealing theory on why I think my life isn't worth living?" His unruffled calm made my want to be spiteful, to shake his composure.

"Your notes tell me very little." He had remained quite unmoved by my vehemence. He was used to dealing with people like me, people who would not bow to the common point of view. But I didn't want to be 'cured'. I wanted to be left alone to die.

I glanced at Dr Stead from under my lowered lids. He was watching me, perfectly still. No doubt he could wait. Rumour had it that some of his patients had been with him five, even ten years. He could wait.

"What makes you so afraid, Miss Thompson?" He repeated, gentle now, concerned.

Instantly I became afraid of my fear. This man paralyzed me. I wanted Dr Christie. I felt I could control him.

"Why can't you just leave me alone? If you left me alone maybe I'd have a chance to get better." The words came in a husky whisper, my sweaty hands clenched, white knuckled, on my knees.

"It's our job as doctors to try and help you feel more positive. And anyway, I don't think you want to be left alone—not really. I wonder Miss Thompson when you will come into the open and be honest with us, with yourself?"

I gave no reply. The silence tolled on between us.

"Well, that's it for today, I'm afraid. I'll be seeing you at the same time each week, meanwhile see if you can work out just why you want to die. What keeps driving you towards suicide. I'm told you were once a very happy person. Oh yes and I'd like you to go to art therapy. Perhaps there you will feel free to express some of your fear."

He rose and went to the door and opened it for me. I was being shown out.

"You can find your own way back?" I nodded and drifted out into the hallway. I wanted desperately to escape, but visions of Angela prevented me from running out in my nightdress. Then, as I looked down the narrow corridor to the main part of the hospital, I saw the outpatients' public phone. I had no money; bed patients were not allowed the independence of money. But a transfer charge call? Surely Dr Christie would accept the cost? He'd understand. The idea settled as a conviction, and I went soundlessly into the booth.

"Enquiries?" I spoke softly, frightened of being caught. I gave the details of Dr. Christie's new hospital, St James, Portsmouth[xxviii] and a minute or two later, the call was put through.

"I have a transfer call on the line for Dr Christie. It's a Clare Thompson calling. Will you pay for the call?"

"Hold on, I'll just check."

A pause and then Christie came on the phone. "Clare? Is that you? What's the matter?" He sounded worried.

"I must see you Dr Christie... Now!... Please." The 'please' was barely audible. It was my way of showing him just how desperate I was. He knew my dread of asking for anything, for revealing even the smallest need, the faintest crack in the armour of self-sufficiency, but I was desperate.

"Where are you, Clare?"

"At Lady Chichester."

"Are you seeing Dr Stead?"

"Yes but..." my throat constricted with emotions I could not express. Why couldn't he just see me?

"Well, I'm afraid that means you're not my patient anymore. I'd have..."

I slammed the receiver down and fled up the stairs to the ward. Turning my head away from the nine pairs of watching eyes I dived under my pillow. He'd rejected me. I had, for the first time, broken and asked him for help and he'd rejected me on a bureaucratic technicality. I started to rock rhythmically, back and forth, back and forth.

Sister Cripps, in charge of the admissions ward, put a hand on the pillow.

"Dr Stead's here to see you, Clare. Sit up." There was a touch of the sergeant major in the command. I clung tighter to my refuge.

"Hello, Miss Thompson. Can you hear me? Dr Christie has just rung. He was worried when you hung up. Can you tell me about it?"

Even through the pillow, I could hear the tension in his voice, the irritation. He no doubt should have been on his way home, back to his wife and family. He had better things to do with his life than cajole sulky twenty-year-olds hiding under pillows.

"Come on!" With an effort he had smoothed the sharp edge out of his voice. "I can't talk to the top of a pillow. I feel such a fool!" He paused. I stopped rocking. "Well, if you really don't want to talk, I'll go home. See you next week." He sounded tired and discouraged.

I heard him walk away down the ward. He must have been reflecting that he had too many patients, and difficult ones at that. 'Sophisticated nuts', as one patient had called us Steadites.

10

To The White House

Sister Cripps put her head round the ward door. "Hannah! Could you take Clare with you when you go down to Art?"

I looked across at my neighbour. Hannah smiled back reassuringly. That day she had applied a particularly exaggerated version of her usual war paint. Black eyeliner stretched from the inner corners of her upper eyelids following their contours, then just under the outer tip of her eyebrows and on to the very extremity of her temples, with another line following the lower lid till the two lines met in a point to form an elongated triangle. She had then smudged her upper eyelids with bruised-purple eyeshadow and filled in the elongated triangle in white.

Growing used to the mask, I was inching my way closer to the person behind it. And, increasingly, I felt drawn to what I found. Hannah, too, was a Steadite with a highly analytical, almost forensic brain and an extraordinarily wide vocabulary which she used very precisely and apparently quite unconsciously.

"Come on Clare, don your robe and let's go."

I wrapped my comforting blue dressing gown around me, and we set off down the stately staircase to the ground floor, our heads together, one dark, one fair.

Art Therapy was held in what must once have been the main drawing room. Rickety black trestle tables stood ranged beneath elaborately moulded cornices and ceiling domes. Bay windows looked out onto the gardens. As we entered, Miss Davies came over, a warm smile offered in welcome. I took to her instantly. Hannah showed me where to find large sheets of white wallpaper lining. Miss Davies handed me pots of poster paints and a selection of brushes.

My first efforts were tentative: a small brush and a cramped design in one corner of the paper. But looking around at the half dozen other patients at work and seeing their wild creations, I grew bolder. Soon I was making sweeping strokes with the best of them, a large brush charged with the pallet's darkest, angriest colours. As I layered one colour thickly over another, one thought on another, some silent spring was released, and I began to paint with fury. Page after page covered in blacks and purples, dark blues and greens, each time a man's face, and then eyes, eyes, eyes. In reds and golds and whites all watching me sadistically. As I finished one, I threw it to the floor and started on another as if some dam had burst. In the silence of the paints, where no words were needed, I'd found release.

"Phew!" said Hannah as we headed upstairs for lunch. "That was impressive. It seemed as if you were really revelling in it!"

"Wasn't it weird? I honestly don't know where it came from, but I suddenly felt burning, fighting anger, black, dark-eyed anger. Do you know, I really think that helped—much more than all this talking stuff."

"Or non-talking stuff in your case," Hannah laughed. It was strange how quickly she and I had clicked. Soulmates in a house full of lost souls.

A few days later, we took ourselves out of the ward and were perched side by side at the top of the stairs, the limits of my unaccompanied freedom until I was given back my clothes.

There, Hannah explained, low-voiced, what had led to her admission. "You see, my father desperately wanted a son. For some people in our faith the firstborn son is far more esteemed than any number of daughters. In fact, do you know what I discovered the other day? Every morning my father stands naked in front of the mirror and thanks God for creating him a man! Can you believe it?" Hannah's voice burned with indignation. "And of course, my poor, deprived father only had us two daughters. But then a miracle occurred. I was fifteen and my sister Rebecca thirteen when, finally, my mother bore him a son. Oh, you should have heard the exultation. '*Barux hashem!* Thank God!'" Hannah raised her hands in mock hosannas. "But they rejoiced too soon, those parents of mine. David had been born with a congenital defect." Hannah paused, gazing into space, remembering.

We sat in silence for a while then Hannah took up her tale again. "Did you know that David means adored in Hebrew? Very apposite, for we did adore him. All of us. He was a minute creature. He never thrived and he cried a lot, but we all loved him, my father most of all." Her voice cracked with emotion. She drew in a deep breath and continued. "And then one day David died. We were all standing around his cot. He'd had a fever. And he just died!" Tears ran down Hannah's cheeks. "And my father—my father gave a heart-rending cry full of pain and turned on me and shouted as if to reach the heavens, 'Why couldn't it have been you? Oh God! Why not you?'"

The cruelty of some parents was beyond belief. How could he? I put out my hand and lightly touched Hannah's arm and held it just long enough to transmit my sympathy but not enough to intrude on her pain. Our friendship was still young.

"I was just sixteen then. Two weeks later I tried to do as he wished: I tried to kill myself. But, yet again, I failed to meet his aspirations. That's when they despatched me to the Bethlem Royal Hospital." A quick pause to give herself time to grab hold of her emotions and ram them back, deep inside. Then Hannah went on in a matter-of-fact voice. "Did you know Bethlem's the oldest lunatic asylum still extant in Europe?[xxix] It's where the word Bedlam comes from." Hannah had once again got herself and her vocabulary tightly under control.

"Clare, would you please keep Belinda company for lunch?" Sister Cripps pulled out a chair beside a small round table placed in the middle of the ward. Once we had our clothes, we would be allowed downstairs to the dining room but, as long as we were in dressing gowns, we had to eat on the ward. Belinda, aged 11, was the hospital's youngest patient. Suffering from anorexia, and weighing almost nothing, they had admitted her to The Lady Chichester in the hopes of avoiding the trauma of being force-fed on the ward of a general hospital.

I looked at this skeleton child with her skeleton wrists sticking out from her dressing gown sleeves, her sunken eyes great pools of wariness, and I longed to hug her, tell her she'd be okay. Belinda had been placed in the middle of the room, the better to keep an eye on her as she ate. They served her a soft diet: mashed potatoes and mince with gravy, puréed vegetables, puréed fruit with custard, to prevent her from squirreling food away. I wondered what my role was supposed to be. Was I the child's jailer? Was I supposed to inform on her as I spotted her trying to slip a spoonful of custard into her dressing gown pocket?

"I wouldn't do that, lovey. Really. You'll make an awful mess. It'll all run down your legs when you stand up."

Belinda looked back at me, her face strained with anxiety and reproach.

"What's it to you what I do?" she whispered. "I've always hated custard."

Suddenly, Mavis, sitting in her wheelchair on the other side of the table, spoke up. "You're going to die, you know, if you go on like that. You have to eat." The words came out in the dull monotone of the deeply depressed.

I looked up, trying to hide my astonishment. It was the first time I'd heard Mavis speak. I had noticed that most of the patients gave her a wide berth, and I had wondered why. Certainly not because she was violent or abusive. Far from it. Perhaps it was because she reminded them all of where they too might end up one day. There was hardly a patient in the place who had not, at some point, contemplated taking their own life. But none of them had had the courage to jump. Mavis was different. Not for her the coward's route to death: pills or razor blades or gas. No, Mavis was in a wheelchair because she had no legs and she had no legs because, when she had thrown herself in front of a train, the train had severed her legs, not her head. Now she was trapped in her body unable to escape, still suicidal but made even more so by the new agony from phantom pains in her phantom legs.

Mavis. The woman in turquoise. Everything about her was turquoise: her nightdress and dressing gown, her slippers, her toothbrush, her face flannel. All in acknowledgement of the fact that she was addicted to that little turquoise pill, sodium amytal. She had been admitted to try and break her addiction but, for Mavis, her life was only made bearable by taking high doses of the medicine. I watched her, wondering if perhaps there was some way I could help. Dared I try to penetrate the silence behind which the middle-aged woman had barricaded herself? Would I be rebuffed?

This lack of outreach on the part on the other patients reminded me of the isolation which meets the newly bereaved when no one dares speak to them, dares ask how they are, for fear they will somehow make the pain worse. Nothing can make the pain worse. A hand held out in empathy can ease it and, indeed, is even more appreciated as the mourner knows what fears such friends have overcome. With all the deaths on the wards when I was nursing, I had learnt to talk calmly to grieving families, to listen to their heartache. Maybe Mavis would like someone, a patient, not a psychoanalyst, to listen to her story.

* * *

"Clare! Dr Stead is ready for you."

Ten days into my stay I wondered what he would have prepared for me this time. Would he bring up my paintings?

He rose to greet me and indicated a chair. "I hear you released a lot of emotion in art therapy. Can you tell me about it? What triggered it?"

"I don't know. I really don't. I was gripped by this great surge of hatred, anger, almost as if I was vomiting it out of me. Hatred for the face on the paper, attacked with the brush, and the paint. They were my weapons. But who was that face? I don't know. I didn't recognise it at all."

Stead sat without moving, alert, listening, waiting for more. He said nothing. I, too, sat and waited. I'd promised to cooperate but the longer I waited the more difficult it became for me to speak. Ten minutes passed like an eternity. Finally, he relented a little.

"Sister tells me you are settling in well, though she mentioned you sometimes cry out in the night. Can you tell me anything about that?"

"Not really. It's something people tell me I've done for months now. I don't know why. I never remember any dreams when I wake up. Just this suffocating fear."

"I gather you also have a problem with closed doors. Have you any idea why *that* is?"

"No. It started during that strange year before I ended up in the York Clinic. Faced with a closed door I sort of became paralysed. Once I was late for a nurses' conference and I waited outside for half an hour before someone else came and opened the door for me. Don't ask me why. I don't know why. I've tried to analyse it. Tried to ask what is it I'm afraid of? What do I think is on the other side of the closed door? Or is it the door itself I'm afraid of? Is it somehow holding me trapped, unable to escape. I don't know."

"Maybe you can tell me something else. You've mentioned you're evil. Do you know why you feel you're evil?"

Evil! Why I feel evil? There are so many different sorts of evil. Cruelty like that shown to Hannah. I don't think I'm cruel. It's something much deeper.

"I don't know. I was first told I was evil by the nuns."

"What nuns?"

"Ursuline nuns in a Belgian convent. It was a strange, repressive place." For the first time I looked Dr Stead in the eye. After all, the story contained nothing intimate at all. "They'd run a hospital for Allied wounded soldiers during the war. Then, after the war, they ran a girls' boarding school. I went there when I was ten. A whole lot of British army brats living in Germany were sent there. Shipped in by the trainload, literally. We were sent in part as a gesture of thanks for the nuns' kindness to our wounded soldiers, partly because it only cost about £50 a term and partly because our parents hoped we'd come out speaking fluent French." I raised my shoulders and one hand in a questioning gesture as I looked at Stead. "What our parents hadn't reckoned with was that the nuns were Catholics whereas we were ninety percent Protestant. Looking back, I think the nuns genuinely saw it as their holy duty to convert us, to save our souls from eternal Purgatory. Anyway, one day one of the nuns, quite a young one, died of a heart attack. And the nun superintending the Middle School, *Les Moyennes,* called all us British Protestant children together and told us we were evil, we'd murdered the nun and that we were all going to burn in everlasting hellfire—unless we converted to Catholicism." I snorted in scorn at such an idea. "But mine's not that sort of evil. I've something dark and fluid inside me, a fermenting essence of evil. Sometimes it almost disappears but it always comes back. I can be feeling fine and then I see it out on the horizon heading like a tidal wave towards me. About to exterminate all those around me. Right now I'm okay."

"Miss Davies from art therapy has suggested that next week you could start over at the White House, the day centre, join in group and art therapy over there. What do you think of that idea?"

"Okay," I replied apathetically whilst, inside, I felt instantly threatened by the very thought of group therapy but, on the other hand, I would finally be allowed my street clothes. Hannah had already been going there for a while. She would show me the ropes.

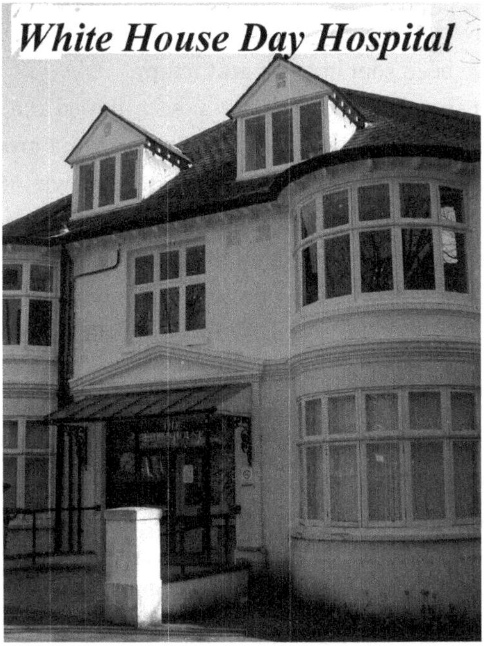

The White House. [Credit: Joe Hughes]

On that first day at the White House, I entered the front door with my breath clutched tight in my throat. Just inside, to the right, a largeish room opened out. I followed Hannah in and sat down close beside her. To my left was a man with pale, sandy hair, thin-faced, nervous. Soon the room filled up with some dozen outpatients, men and women whose ages ranged from eighteen to somewhere in their sixties. They came in daily from the surrounding town. Only Hannah and I were inmates from the Chich.

As the meeting started, the psychiatric social worker, John Patten, introduced me and then asked the other patients to introduce themselves. Some were relaxed, open, even joking whilst others were barely able to mutter their names. I sympathised. I sat rigid, my hands clenched, awaiting the inevitable moment when I would have to speak. When, at the end of the introductions, I was asked to say a few words, my mind went a complete blank. What was I supposed to say?

"I don't know. I'm twenty. I'm a patient across the road in The Lady Chichester. I've been sent here for art therapy."

For the first few days they left me alone, allowed me to settle in. I was afraid. What might they uncover? I studied the group dynamics. Here were patients with mindsets similar to my own. Might they not recognise the ploys and deceits that I hid behind? Some were trying to help but others were out to demolish, to divert attention away from themselves and their own chaos by exposing others. John Patten acted as umpire but wouldn't he, too, want to use questions to prise open the blackness that I guarded so fiercely?

Saying nothing at all clearly opened one to being questioned. I decided the best strategy was to make several small contributions at each meeting, all sweet, kind, concerned, helpful, so as not to antagonise anyone which, in turn, might lead to their retaliation.

The group was basically divided into those who wanted to talk about themselves and their problems and those, like myself, who didn't want to be there at all. My strategy was to draw out the talkers, hoping that they would, between them, fill the whole two-hour session. Overall, it worked pretty well. I began to get to know the others and to feel more comfortable. Colin, the guy who had been beside me the first day, became a friend. A quiet man some ten years my senior, he was a keen photographer and a gentle companion, occasionally asking me to pose for innocent photos on the White House lawn.

Then one day a new patient turned on me.

"So, Clare, you said you tried to kill yourself. How come it didn't work?" He sounded like my first doctor. It felt like a case conference! I felt the rest of the group tense, watch me to see how I would react, some of them ready to join the man now that my invisible, protective wall had been breached. Holding myself in check, my voice languid and cool as a moonlit pool, I replied, "I was just unlucky, I guess."

"But it's not a question of luck. It's a question of organization and guts. Didn't you have the guts to hang yourself? Was that it?"

"And how about you, Graham? Have you never had the fortitude to cast yourself from a bridge?" Hannah had leapt to my rescue. The tension in the room mounted. The focus switched on to the new man, Graham.

11

Assault, Booze and Therapy

NOW ALLOWED MY street clothes, I could go down to the town or the beach whenever I wanted. The afternoon had turned cold and blustery. Telling Sister Cripps I was going for a walk on the promenade, I collected my anorak from the coat cupboard and set out alone. Grey clouds scudded across the horizon. The wind snatched at my hair and tugged at my jacket. What joy to be alone, buffeted by the elements, watching as the fuming waves rolled in to crash upon the shingle, their sibilant hissing soothing to my ears.

My mind must have been far away as I leant against the railing, gazing out to sea, for I didn't notice the man until he was right next to me, tugging at my sleeve. I looked round surprised, half fearful. Why hadn't I heard him? The wind and the waves must have masked his approach. He brought his stubbled face close to mine. His hands trembled. His eyes looked pleading, as if he was about to cry. The next moment he grabbed me, fumbling with his fly, pushing me up against the railings, pressing himself against me, rubbing his engorged penis up and down, up and down against my trousers and jerking off.

But I wasn't there. I'd already fled to that cool secret place that I'd discovered at some point in a mislaid past. I searched myself for panic but there was none. No fear of being touched. Nothing. But why? Was it because I was numbed? Was it the anguish in his face? The desperation? The lack of aggression? Was it the feeling that in some way he wasn't a stranger, he was sick, one of us? Was that why I found him so sad?

A police car cruised by bringing me back to earth. I thought of hailing them but paused, and then did nothing. Instead, I turned on the man, suddenly incensed, yelling, almost as a mother might yell at her child after he'd run into the road.

"Are you crazy? I could have handed you in then! You'd have been in *big* trouble! You *are* in big trouble. You need to see someone and soon or you're going to end up in jail... You're damned lucky it was me you attacked and not someone else."

"I know! I know, I know!" the man broke in, his voice pitiful, shaking. "I'm sorry! I'm so sorry. I can't help it. I get driven. I can't stop it. I don't know what to do. Here take this. Please!"

He pulled a wad of bank notes out of his pocket and thrust them at me.

"I don't want it!" I snapped, batting his hand away. "Give it to charity! And get yourself a psychiatrist. If you don't know one, go to the White House up the far end of the promenade. Someone there will help you."

"Thank you! Thank you so much. I'm so sorry!" And he turned towards the town, head drawn down between his hunched shoulders, hastening away.

Was this the trigger that, several days later, sent me down to the seafront and into an off licence?

"What can I do for you, young lady?"

"I'd like half a bottle of whisky." The man looked at me questioningly, but I was clearly over eighteen so there was not much he could do. I paid, picked up the bottle wrapped in its brown paper bag and walked out without a backward glance. I had decided to 'drown my sorrows'. The promenade had a number of benched shelters looking out to sea. With it being November I was unlikely to be disturbed. I chose a protected corner in one of the shelters, pulled the paper bag open enough to unscrew the cap and took a swig. I almost puked. I had always hated liquor. Couldn't bear the taste—nor the sensation come to that. Maybe I'd made a mistake. Maybe I should have chosen gin or vodka? But it was whisky that I had and whisky it would have to be.

I don't know how long I'd been sitting on the bench drinking methodically from my paper bag, when a man sat down near me. I looked at him through wavering eyes.

"D'yer wan' a drink?" I asked, brandishing the paper bag in his direction.

The man looked at me, puzzled. "*Pardon?* I do not understand. I am French. Please say again."

I looked at him earnestly and tried hard to bring my lips and tongue under control enough to speak clearly.

"I ashed, d'yer wan' a drink? Is that why you've sat here? To drink my whishky?" And I pulled the bottle out of the bag and showed it to him. To my surprise it was already three quarters empty. "You wan' some?"

"Oh no! *Non merci!*" And the poor man got up and walked swiftly away.

I returned to the bottle. It might be disgusting but it seemed to be doing the job. I couldn't really feel anything at all now. Desolation drowned.

Bottle empty, I got unsteadily to my feet and staggered towards the pebble beach. I would go for a swim. But as my tottering feet came in contact with the kerb leading up to the beach I tripped and crashed to the ground, dropped the bottle and lay still.

Slowly I became aware that I needed to find a public lavatory. I needed a pee, and I was probably going to throw up. I managed to raise myself on hands and knees and then with a huge effort stood upright. Triumphant. I felt quite proud of myself. I headed back towards the promenade where I could see a public convenience. But again, I missed the kerb and once more collapsed earthwards. This time pain flared up from both knees. I put my hands down to feel them and my hands came away red with gore. I looked at them in wonder.

Back on my feet again, I now wove my way successfully to my destination. There I threw up mightily, peed and then went to the sink to see what I could do about the blood. It was while I was trying ineffectually to wash it away that a smartly dressed, middle-aged woman stepped in. She looked at me in consternation.

"My dear! What have you done? You poor thing. That looks terrible! Just you wait there while I call an ambulance. Don't move. I'll be back very soon."

While she was gone, I returned to the lavatory, vomited some more and then came out and scooped up water to wash out my mouth. My head was swirling so I sat down on the floor, leant back against the wall and waited.

I came to as the woman returned with two ambulance men. Whilst the woman watched protectively from afar, they examined my knees, washed them with disinfectant and then bandaged them up temporarily before helping me to my feet and, between them, steering me to the ambulance. I tried to thank the woman, but my tongue failed to cooperate.

"Right, love, so where do you live?" The ambulance driver sounded friendly.

"Th'funny farm."

"And what do you mean by that then?"

"I mean th'funny farm. Nut'ouse. Loony bin. God! You know, the Lady Chich."

The guys looked at each other and kept on course for the nearest emergency department. There the staff undid the bandages, swabbed the area down, neatly cut away strands of trailing flesh and then bandaged both knees up again. Next came an anti-tetanus jab. They told me the blood test showed I'd drunk around 10 shots of whisky. Up in the ward, they shifted me from the trolley to a bed, pulled up the cot sides so I couldn't fall out and left me to sleep it off.

I woke late the next morning with a raging thirst and a splitting headache and huge bandages on my knees. It took me a while to work out where I was, and even longer to remember why. Later two nurses turned up to take me back to The Lady Chichester.

That afternoon Dr Stead called by my bed. "How do you feel now?" he asked, his usually neutral voice warmed by sympathy.

"I'm okay," I murmured faintly.

"Clare, couldn't you have told someone, Sister or me, that things were getting bad again?"

I turned away and silently shook my head.

"Well, I'll leave you now, but we'll talk about it some more at our next meeting." And he reached his hand out, patted my bedcover reassuringly and left.

Next morning I hobbled across the road to the White House knowing full well that this time there would be no escape. This time I couldn't shield myself with sweet words from the groups' prying questions.

"So, Clare, what can you tell us about yesterday?" John Patten spoke quite gently but clearly would brook no evasion.

"Nothing much. I went out and got bloody drunk." A ripple of laughter went around the room.

Colin cut in. "Hey, why didn't you tell me? I would have come too."

Another man piped up. "What have yer done to yer knees, ducks? Yer looks like a likely runner for the 4.30!" Again the group laughed, a warm, friendly, enfolding laugh. I relaxed. I would probably survive.

"But that doesn't explain why you wanted to get drunk in the first place, does it?" I should have guessed John Patten wasn't going to let me off that lightly.

"I was in search of oblivion. I wanted to drown my sorrows. You read about it in books. I thought I'd see if it worked."

"And did it?"

I paused. Yes, in a way it did. That terrible need for punishment, that burden of guilt and shame that had to be assuaged. Yes, I had hurt myself. I had punished myself.

"Yes. I feel calmer now. I feel I can breathe again."

The whisky had, momentarily, expunged the need for punishment—that moral duty to die. My spirits rose, indeed neared euphoria, as energy returned. Suddenly life seemed flushed with colour. It tinted the sun yellow and the sea blue, where before everything had been that monochrome grey of the deeply depressed.

The next day, while everyone else was in the day room having coffee, I crept silently up to the art room. I found a long paint brush and some black ink. I climbed onto a chair and slowly covered one whole, pristine white wall with a quote that had been haunting me. A quote from Soren Kierkegaard, the Danish existentialist philosopher.

"Only when a man has become so unhappy and has grasped the misery of this existence so profoundly that he can truly say 'For me Life is worthless', only then can Life have worth in the highest degree."

It was my message of hope, my gift to the inhabitants of the White House.

* * *

Somehow, one piece of rebellion led to another.

"Hannah, what do you say? Shall we run away? Take a trip to London? They can't stop us! After all we may be under-age, but we're not Sectioned. My brain's crying out from boredom. Let's *do* something!"

We were sitting in the hospital garden. Hannah, smoking a cigarette, looked up surprised and searched my face, no doubt wondering what crazy fire was eating me now.

"If you like. Do you think we can achieve it?" she asked in her strangely controlled way. "We'd have to plan it meticulously. When's your next appointment with Stead?"

We put our heads together to plot. We'd need money for the train. That was okay. We could take out some of our sickness benefit from the post office and I still had some savings from my frugal years as a nurse. I would take along my cheque book just in case.

The station was quite a walk from the hospital. We decided to time it. Next, we had to pick a day. Saturday seemed the best. There was no group therapy at weekends. We could go out after breakfast, tell the staff we were off for a walk along the beach. No one would miss us until lunch, by which time we should be well on our way.

The walk to the station took almost 45 minutes. There we picked up a timetable to study the London trains. We called in at the post office and withdrew part of our savings. If we were quick, we could finish breakfast by 8.45am and leave at 9am. (It would look suspicious if we went for a walk along the promenade too early.) That meant we'd arrive at the station around 9.45am. Buy a cheap day return and catch the 9.50 train arriving at Victoria Station around 10.30.

If it hadn't been for sedatives neither of us would have slept that night, the prospect of adventure burnt so brightly. And make no mistake, for patients in The Lady Chichester, an unaccompanied train journey, without permission, was an adventure of the highest order.

At the station we queued for tickets, nervously glancing around the concourse, fearful of being spotted by a member of staff before we'd even passed 'Go'.

Once on the train we began to relax. I watched, mesmerised, as the world rushed by beyond the window, so different to my other life, the one that was draining me, drip by slothful drip, to oblivion. Could I ever reach out and drag myself back to this life in the fast lane?

I felt the excitement rising, my cheeks flushed with hope. Suddenly being alive—and young—was not so bad! I had donned my most flamboyant and most mini of skirts for this foray into the capital while Hannah, dressed as always in black, had taken exceptional care with her make-up.

As the train pulled into Victoria Station we got up, partners in crime, brushed down what there was of our skirts and looked at each other half-scared, half-exultant We'd done it! We'd made it to London.

"Come on, Hannah!" I cried excitedly. "What shall we do first?"

"Carnaby Street! Let's go window shopping, right the way from top to bottom!"

"Okay! We better take the Tube. Oxford Circus's the nearest station."

Oxford Circus. Abruptly memories of degradation and misery flashed into my consciousness, but I fought back, thrusting the images down into that dark abyss from where they'd come.

As we strode down Regent Street, I watched my reflection in the shop windows, for the first time admiring my calf-hugging, almost knee-high black suede, lace-up boots. They looked okay, as did my long expanse of well-turned leg. Startled, I realised that I actually felt good about myself. Was it for the first time ever?

"Come on," I said. "Let's get there before lunch."

Arriving at the Carnaby Street sign, we marvelled at the psychedelic buildings neatly echoing my psychedelic miniskirt. We turned to each other and laughed. And for once, the laughter reached Hannah's eyes. We swaggered off, on top of the world. For a moment we felt we belonged. Maybe we weren't outcasts after all, we were just orbiting in the wrong space. Not weird, just hip! Not unacceptable nutcases but, in an offbeat way, genuine paid-up members of the Swinging Sixties.

"I don't know about you but I'm starving! You know what I'd really like to do? Go to that 360° panoramic restaurant I read about, you know, high up in the Hilton overlooking Hyde Park!"

"Do you think they would permit us to enter? We're not very presentable."

"I don't know. I think we're okay. Let's be brave! Let's give it a try."

The intimidatingly elegant woman at reception coolly directed us to the lifts and told us to get out at the 28th floor. We were early. The maître d' himself ushered us to a table for two, set back just one row from the renowned window, below which stretched much of London.

The menu arrived and we looked at it in shock. I had never realised that food could cost so much. I reassured Hannah, "Don't worry, I've got my cheque book, but we'd better stick to two courses."

I chose rare steak with chips and green salad. How long was it since I'd eaten a really good steak, one that melted in the mouth like mousse? And chips were never found on psychiatric hospital menus. they'd have become flabby long before they reached the table. Hannah went for plaice with prawns, also items seriously missing in our canteen diet. For pudding we both chose fresh fruit salad and cream.

We were just waiting for our first course to arrive when in walked a family group which headed straight for the large, reserved, oval table in the window. I watched them intently. There seemed to be two sets of parents, three children and an extra female. Raptly eavesdropping, I discovered in admiration that everyone, including the children, seemed able to switch effortlessly, in mid-sentence, between three languages. English and French were easily recognisable but what was the third? I turned to Hannah and whispered "What do you think the other language is? It's not Italian, its not sing-songy enough. It's not Portuguese either, that's more nasal." It wasn't until the family left that the woman bringing up the rear, possibly a governess, leant over, smiled and mouthed to me, "Greek!"

Asking for the bill, I noticed a slight twitch of an eyebrow from the maître d' as I pulled out my upmarket Coutts cheque book. Due to some benefactor, all the nurses at the Middlesex Hospital automatically qualified for an exclusive Coutts bank account. I signed a cheque for what seemed a frighteningly large amount of money to cover a two-course lunch with water.

Getting up to leave, we went first to the great window that overlooked Hyde Park, designed as a pleasure garden in the 16th century by Henry

VIII himself. There, in the distance, was the Serpentine Lake, popular with hundreds of thousands of visitors each year. Looking down 28 floors to the street far below, it crossed my mind that maybe here was the ultimate answer: break the window and jump.

"Hey! Look! What's that crowd?" Hannah interrupted my thoughts, pointing to the top of Park Lane.

"Golly, that must be Speakers' Corner! Come on! Let's see what's happening! Could be it's a demo!"

Leaving the hotel, we took off briskly through the park while I recounted to Hannah some of the quirky types I'd met in the past at the Corner.

"I often used to come here on my summer Sundays off. It was terrific entertainment, and all for free, listening to all the crazy views being spouted and relishing the freedom that enshrines our right to do so." I was on a roll, taken out of myself and the recent past, and back to happier times when I had felt young, uninhibited and alive. For a second it crossed my mind that maybe I was manic-depressive.

"I remember one old man, roughly dressed, standing on his black soap box. He was hilarious and he drew a big crowd. He went on and on about how all the men in the crowd wearing jackets were hypocrites, because under their jackets they had holes in their shirts! He kept challenging them to take their jackets off. But no one did! Which, he claimed, just proved his point. But the men kept shouting witty ripostes, all in great good humour. People could say anything!"

By now we had reached the crowd that stretched back from a wooden stage into the park itself. In a newfound high of bravado, I forced a path to the front with Hannah close behind. A man was haranguing the people and then I saw a huge banner proclaiming "BILLY GRAHAM", the famous American Evangelist.

As the realisation struck home, the man on the stage called out in resonating tones, "Now let us bow our heads in prayer!"

Hannah looked at me, her eyes wide with terror, her body frozen. Swiftly my friend's problems flashed through my mind like strobe light warnings: claustrophobic... fear of being looked at... of being trapped... Jewish stuck in a crowd of praying Christians... Why hadn't I thought?

Grabbing Hannah's wrist, I bent forward as if my head was a battering ram and beat a retreat, dragging my friend after me. Ignoring the bowed heads, we shoved and dodged. Some looked up and glared. We finally made it to open ground where, knees shaking, we sank together onto the grass. For a while we said nothing, each unscrambling our own conflicted emotions.

Underneath the buzz of adrenalin and the euphoria of rebellion, the day had already taken its toll on me. We looked at each other, drained and weary.

"I think it's time to withdraw," said Hannah. I almost caught myself adding, 'back home'.

The return journey passed in silence, each gazing sightless out of the window, thoughts turned inwards, trying to assess the damage done, the fragile, dandelion seeds of confidence so swiftly blown away. We were also missing our medication. I dug my fingers into my aching arm. Despite all the planning, I'd forgotten I'd be without my DF118.

We arrived back at The Chich in time for supper, our spirits momentarily revived thanks to the enthusiastic reception from our friends. The punishment was mild: grounded for forty-eight hours, our street clothes locked away. We agreed it could have been worse. Meanwhile our shared adventure, shared history, meant that the bond between us had grown ever stronger.[xxx]

12

Signing Out

WE PREPARED TO face the music in the White House, but it turned out that people were more interested in hearing of our brief adventure than in trying to analyse why we'd done it. After all, that was pretty obvious.

The following day I entered Stead's office in trepidation. What would he say? How would he interpret our actions according to Saint Freud? God how I hated Freud! Twisting and turning everything one said or did to mean something else, everyone dancing to the tunes of his id, his ego and his superego. The guy had clearly sat gazing at his own navel for far too long—and then turned the crud that he'd found there into some universal truth.

In the event Dr Stead didn't even try an interpretation.

"Come in Miss Thompson. Do sit down. Tell me, was it fun?" And his blue, knowing eyes smiled at me in amusement. Could it be he was actually proud of our escapade? Even saw it as healthy?

"Yes. Yes it was! At least most of the time."

"And what about the rest?"

"I don't know. I think it was all too much. You know it's easy to become institutionalised in here. To forget how to carry on outside. Then there was the Billy Graham crowd. I should never have dragged Hannah into it. I didn't think!

"What did you do?"

"We ran away as fast as we possibly could."

"Tell me something, Miss Thompson." Stead's tone had changed. "When are you going to stop running away from yourself—and me?"

I paused, then looking my psychiatrist in the eye, replied, "When there's nowhere left to run to."

We sat on in silence.

A few weeks later, Hannah was discharged back to her parents. I was devastated. We had become so close, soul mates, sisters. In times of stress we instinctively understood where each was coming from. I felt the loss of Hannah even more deeply than that of Roland. Yet another abandonment. Like my childhood when I was constantly moving schools, having to say goodbye to friends. But we kept in touch with frequent letters until one day I learnt that Hannah had found a boyfriend, had left her parents and moved in with him. She had separated herself from Loony Land—at least for a while.

* * *

As my twenty-first birthday approached, I felt more and more trapped. From the beginning I had sworn to myself that the day I turned twenty-one I would sign my discharge papers. Like so many of the mentally troubled, I had a deep intolerance of those who did not keep their word. I had made a promise to myself so now I had to keep it, however exhausted and battered I felt. Waves of blackness loomed on the horizon as I planned to cut the umbilical cord that attached me to the strange haven that was The Lady Chich. In a few weeks I would legally be able to vote, to refuse treatment, to take control of my life. Only now I wasn't sure I knew how. What if I couldn't make it in the outside world? What if I failed yet again? What then?

Feeling doomed but determined, I started scanning the local newspaper for jobs. I spotted one for a dishwasher in a factory kitchen on the local industrial estate and then an advertisement for a bedsit in a private home nearby. Telling no one, I applied for the factory job and got an appointment. My plan was to take The Chich by surprise on my birthday so that nothing could stop my discharge.

Arriving at the factory premises, I looked at the large prefab and saw a door. A closed door. But I had to knock on it. On the other side my future boss might be waiting. I knocked. A man opened the door. "Clare Thompson?" I smiled nervously and nodded. "I'm Jim Stewart from personnel." He held out his hand. "Come on in. I see you trained as a nurse. I'm curious. What made you apply for this job? Have you ever done anything like it before?"

"No, no I haven't. I've been off work for a while. I found nursing too depressing. I thought this would suit me better."

The man considered me for a moment, taking in what I had—and had not—said. "Well, it's very easy. Come and let's take a look." He led me down a corridor and opened the door into a vast kitchen. "Here's where you'll be. All the cleaned crockery gets dipped in these vats of boiling water for sterilising and then the racks are pulled out onto here and then each cup is dried and stacked over there. There's usually four or five other women working in here." He crossed the room. "And this," he said with a touch of excitement in his voice. "This is our new machine for peeling potatoes! All you have to do is feed it from these sacks and then take the peeled potatoes over to the chef. Amazing! The actual canteen's here." He took me to some swing doors, glass-portholes in the top half. I peered through at row upon row of tables and chairs stretching into the distance. *Thank God I don't have to go in there.*

"After lunch you help clean the cafeteria, all the kitchen machinery, then brush, mop and disinfect the floor and dry it with another mop. Once that's done you can sign out. Oh and these are the disposable caps that all our kitchen staff have to wear. Hygiene and all that. And that's about it. Simple really. What do you think?"

I glanced around. It certainly looked easy enough. It fitted in with my ambitions too: anonymity, obscurity, a job that could be done without having to think. And I would earn enough to get by. I agreed to start work the Monday after my birthday.

Next, I went in search of the bedsit I'd seen advertised. It reminded me of that other life, so long ago, when I had also gone searching for a house. A house owned by a woman who told me I was going to go mad. This latest home proved to be up a typical suburban street lined with decorative trees and with a pleasant little neighbourhood park.

The woman who came to the door was short with a kind, apple-cheeked round face, and was drying her hands on her apron as if she might have been doing the washing-up. She looked at me enquiringly.

"I've come about the bedsit. I read about it in the paper. I've just signed up for a job on the estate."

The woman's face relaxed. "Wonderful! Do come on in. I'll show you round. I'm Mary." And she held out her hand.

"And my name's Clare, Clare Thompson." I took the proffered hand before following the woman upstairs.

"So, here's the bedroom. It's not very big I'm afraid but the bed's comfy and here, next door, this is the bathroom. We share that but there's only meself and me son in the house now. Me husband died. That's why I'm having to let out the rooms. Can't afford to keep the house otherwise. And then here's your little kitchen."

It was certainly little, but I fell in love with it instantly. There was a tall window looking down the narrow back garden, a small pine table against the wall with three light pine kitchen chairs and, opposite, a sink, a double electric hob and simple, fitted, pine cupboards on the wall above. I felt a flicker of pleasure warm inside me. It would all be mine. I didn't have to share it with anyone. My kingdom, my space.

"Where are you living now?" Mary asked.

I paused. Should I lie? But Mary wasn't 'staff', wasn't part of the psychiatric conglomerate. I could not lie to her.

"I'm at The Lady Chichester Hospital right now but I'll be discharged shortly."

"The Lady Chich?" and the woman beamed up at me. "Isn't that a coincidence! I was there. After me husband died you know. They were ever so good to me. Oh, I'll be happy to have you taking the rooms. When can you move in?"

* * *

And so the big day came. The day I'd once so longed for, the day I now dreaded. As soon as Sister Cripps came on duty, I asked to speak to her in her office. There I looked her in the eye and said, "I'm twenty-one today. I need the forms. I've come to discharge myself."

"I know Clare. I know. Congratulations! But *you* know you're not ready, love. Not quite yet." Sister Cripps looked at me anxiously. Was she crestfallen? Did she feel she'd somehow failed? Of course, all good psychiatric nurses hope their patients will get better, come to a truce with their pasts and the world and go out courageously to meet their future. And *not* return. No doubt she and Dr Stead had long foreseen the possibility of me demanding to be discharged, had probably even discussed whether they had the right to stop me. To Section me.

Even as I asked, I knew I would never survive out there for long. Not now. Surely I had learnt that from my London fiasco? Did Sister, with her long experience perhaps sense that I didn't really want to go? Was my fear, lurking beneath my brash surface, as palpable to her as it was to me? Fear that I would fail, be dragged back inside and locked up for ever. It was almost as if signing out was another way of destroying myself.

"Where are you going to go? What will you do for money?"

"I've found a job and a bedsit. I'll manage. I just need a repeat prescription for my arm."

"Clare, please don't do it! You're still not well. Really. It's hard, hard, hard for patients out there."

"I know. Hannah's out there. I've seen. But I'm 21. I've got the right to discharge myself. I want the papers. I want to sign them now."

Reluctantly, Sister Cripps went to the bureau and pulled out a form. She sat me down at an old-fashioned *escritoire* in front of the window. A window that looked out over the gardens where patients who wished could hoe and plant and water, could nourish the earth and create new life. I, too, had been, in my way, nourished and cared for. But I knew I mustn't think of that, and I turned my attention firmly to the form. First Sister Cripps filled in her part at the top, then I mine and then Dr Stead was called in to give the final signature and to write me up for a month's medication.

I was free to leave.

I went back to the ward to collect the new hold-all that I'd bought, then returned to the office to say a restrained goodbye to the two people who, over the past months, I knew had done their best to help me. Dr Stead shook my hand. "Best of luck, Miss Thompson."

Sister Cripps momentarily held my hands in hers, gave them a reassuring squeeze and said, "Can I help you with your bag?"

"No, no thank you, I can manage." I smiled rather wistfully, picked up the bag and as Dr Stead put a light hand on my shoulder, headed for the door.

"If you ever need us, you know where we are," he said, holding the door open for me.

I walked down the drive and across the road to the bus stop.

With my birthday falling on a Friday, the family had decided to drive down on the Saturday for a celebratory meal by the sea. John's twenty-first had been held with much pomp at The Rag, our father's London Club; Dave's with just the family at Prunier's, a famous London fish restaurant. I frankly dreaded the whole fuss but knew it to be inescapable. I decided not to mention I had already left The Chich. Lunch was going to be difficult enough as it was.

I deliberately arrived a little early at Brighton's Old Ship Hotel and, picking up a newspaper, moved to a deep, leather-upholstered armchair at the far end of the lobby to calm myself for what was to come. Just after one o'clock the whole family was scooped, one by one, through the rotating wooden doors and deposited into reception. I rose to greet them. Each gave me a hug, showing various degrees of warmth, and rather too heartily congratulated me. They swapped their coats for numbered tickets, and we headed for the dining room.

Two tables at the far end were occupied. The rest of the room was a sea of starched white linen with large napkins, pleated like fans, standing rigid in the centre of each place setting. Our reserved table already had champagne flutes waiting for the celebration to begin. *Thank goodness for champagne. Should ease the tension.* As the family went to their places each one delivered a wrapped present onto my place setting.

When the wine waiter arrived to uncork the Moët & Chandon and fill the flutes I placed a hand over mine. My adventures with the whisky had turned me teetotal, indeed just a whiff of alcohol now made me feel ill.

"Go on Clare," said John. "Open your presents. Let's see what you've got!" I hated opening presents in front of other people. What if I didn't like them? Was I supposed to lie and say that I did? Give a great big smile of joy that was only lip deep?

I picked up the bulky one from my mother first as I was pretty sure I knew what was inside. Wrapped in her favourite colour, blue, the paper was patterned with Monet's waterlilies. Out of habit, I carefully undid the creamy ribbon holding the packet together and then the paper so it could all be neatly folded and used again. Sure enough, there was just the outfit I had asked for. All in black. Was it Hannah's influence? It was a huge relief to be able to get up and give my mother a great big hug. I held up the mini-kilt and swirled around to show everyone. Next came John's present: Joan Baez and Bob Dylan LPs. I felt my face light up. "John, they're wonderful. I love them already."

Dave's present was in a small box wrapped in black tissue paper: the prettiest pair of gold earrings shaped like petalled flowers with a real pearl at the centre of each. I took them out of their cushioned silk and screwed them onto my ear lobes and turned my head back and forth for all to see.

And so only my father's present remained. Unwrapping it slowly, I prayed I would like that too. A book, I knew from its shape, but what book? As I lifted it out, my eyes filled with tears as they swept over it and my hands tenderly caressed its beauty. For it was more than a work of art, it was a work of love. My father had bound a book just for me. It was a 1735 edition of the comedy, *The Careless Husband*, by C Cibber. On the outside, bound in sky blue leather, he had engraved an actor's mask and below it had put my initials, CT, and the year 1964, all picked out in gold leaf. But why 1964? Was it a mistake? After all, it was now 1967. Or was it a hint that I should return to my dream of acting, a dream that had indeed flourished—and died—in 1964?

"Oh Dad! But that's beautiful! Just beautiful! Thank you so much!" I put my arms around him as he sat beside me and gave him a lingering embrace. My father and I had never been very good at talking to each other. I didn't share things with him like I did with my mother, but I always knew that he loved me and that I loved him. It was only when I opened the book that I found a very handsome cheque for two hundred pounds lying inside. (Enough today to buy an elderly second hand car.)[xxxi]

His present reminded me of how proud I had been when, aged eight, he had given me the complete works of John Keats for Christmas. Poetry was my great treat on the Sundays when he was home. He would stand, tall and gently handsome, one arm resting on the mantelpiece in the drawing room and read Keats' poems to me in his mellifluous, velvet voice. My favourite was *Ode to a Nightingale*. I loved its sad cadences. Thinking of Keats in turn made me think of Roland and his present of the works of Shelley. I wondered where Roland was now. How he was coping?

"So, who's going to propose the toast? Dad?" John broke in on my thoughts.

Dad stood up. He raised his glass and smiled wistfully at me, his only daughter. "It is with great pleasure that I propose a toast to our dear Clare on the occasion of her coming of age, and to her future which I am sure will soon shine brightly again. Please stand and raise your glasses. To Clare!" My family rose and repeated in unison, "To Clare!"

Then, before they could sit down, he carried on, "And now to our ancient toast: To absent friends."

I stood to join them, empty glass in hand, and, as a family, we repeated our annual Christmas toast, "To Absent Friends and all friends round St Pauls." Then we clinked our glasses together to fend off the evil spirits. I looked around in wonder. That traditional toast, known to Dickens and many others, had somehow, all on its own, overcome our recent divisions, brought us together as a family, standing together against adversity. After they'd sipped their Moët & Chandon, we sat down. Then, quite suddenly, a lost memory came flooding back, one yet to be re-posted on my memory wall. Moët & Chandon! Of course!

I turned, animated, to John and then my parents. "It's just come back! Moët & Chandon. Do you remember? That first time we went there? I was twelve. We were supposed to be staying in a flat in Paris, just you Mum, and Dad and me. And then the owner of the flat got German measles and couldn't go away so instead she introduced us to a friend of hers, Moira Campbell, who was the hostess at the Chandon chateau, what was it called? You know, John."

"Saran, Chateau de Saran."

"That's it! You went there later, didn't you? Worked as a tourist guide in the cellars in the holidays from university or something. And we had bottles of champagne by our bath and huge white fluffy towels, do you remember, Mum?" I turned to my mother, eyes wide and alight with the newfound memory.

"And wonderful sloping views down across the vineyards."

"And the dinner! I'll never forget the dinner. We sat at a big round table with some other guests, all adults. There was a menu which was passed round. And then there was this terrible cheese soufflé brought by the butler. At least, it was delicious but serving it was a nightmare. The cheese was all sort of stringy, a bit like trying to help yourself to spaghetti, and I kept pulling and pulling, trying to get a detached spoonful onto my plate. I felt so embarrassed, sure everyone was watching me."

"Yes," Mum chimed in. "I remember looking across the table and seeing you struggling!"

"And do you remember the water? Moira must have realised I didn't drink wine, so she asked the butler to bring me a glass of water. And I looked at the water, paralysed. What was I supposed to do with it?" I now turned to the others to explain. "Do you remember back then, everyone in England was warned never to drink the water in France? Moira, sensing my confusion, sent the butler to explain to you, Mum, that it was okay to drink. But you didn't understand him. And she didn't realise I spoke French."

"Heavens, how do you remember all that?" my mother asked.

"I don't know. It just came to me, that and the huge, warm, cuddly bath towels. Real luxury! I loved it there."

Tensions broken, the meal continued in much happier vein with innumerable reminiscences and counter-reminiscences as we each recalled family events differently, accused each other of making stories up and laughing. *Maybe this party isn't such a bad thing after all. I can't remember when I last saw Mum and Dad looking so relaxed.* Eventually we all got up to leave. Dad suggested they drop me off at The Lady Chich. I paused, daring myself to tell them I'd left. But then, ducking out, not wanting to break the warmth of our reconciliation, I replied, "No, it's okay, I've a few things I need to do. Thank you so much and thank you all for a wonderful lunch and wonderful presents!"

Collecting their coats, we enjoyed final embraces before the rest of the family went off to retrieve Dad's car.

I sat and waited a while before picking up my gifts, bundling them into one of the carrier bags and making my way to the bus stop from where a bus would carry me to my new home.

13

Free?

MONDAY MORNING. As I tentatively pushed open the factory kitchen door, a barrage of eyes swivelled towards me, middle-aged eyes. I must have been the only one there under forty. I stood stock still as they scrutinised me. Assessed me? Judged me? Then one woman broke away from the pack and came over, smiling.

"'Ello! Come on in! I'm Pat. Are you the new girl, Clare?"

I nodded.

"Mr Stewart told me to keep an eye out for yer." Pat was around my mother's age, with an ample figure and a kind, rumpled face. "Come with me, ducks, and we can hang your things up. 'Ere we go," and she opened a metal wardrobe and handed me a hanger for my coat and handbag. "'Ere's yer overall. Nice blue, I reckon, what d'yer think?"

"Lovely. I love blue." And I felt my smile almost reach my anxious eyes.

"So, you'll start off each mornin' stickin' the clean plates out in the canteen ready for dinner. You just grab them from those stacks and take 'em through there." Pat pointed to the canteen's swing door.

The plates weighed a ton, making me realise how pathetically weak I'd become from months of inaction. Soon my arm was screaming out at me, and I wondered when I could take a break for some more DF118. I felt embarrassed swallowing them in public. Eventually I had some 150 plates stacked neatly in the cafeteria's serving area.

Next came loading the potatoes into the fancy new machine. Scared I'd do it wrong, I turned to my mentor.

"Sorry, Pat, Mr Stewart did show me, but could you show me again just exactly what I have to do?"

"Sure." Pat gave a swift and simple demonstration after which I soon got the hang of it. By the end I was actually feeling quite chuffed with how the morning was going. At least I hadn't disgraced myself yet.

Then it was time for lunch.

"Come on, Clare, time to help serve up the dinner."

"What! Mr Stewart said my work was all in the kitchen. That's what the advert said too. That's why I signed up."

"Hmmm, that's odd. Don't know why Mr Stewart told yer that. Sorry, mate, but everyone has to help at dinner time. It's part of the job. It's not bad. They're nice enough fellers out there. Probably take the mick a bit to begin with, what with yer posh accent and yer being so young an' all, but once they get used to yer they'll treat you right. Come on now!"

Very reluctantly I followed Pat through the swing doors, my pulse already racing in alarm. The canteen was rapidly filling up with men.

"Hey lovey! What's yer name then?" one man called out.

"Clare."

"Hey George, did yer 'ear that! Say that again, love, so George can 'ear yer."

I flinched, tried to drown my middle-class accent and said more loudly, "Clare."

"Cor blimey, where d'yer come from? Not around 'ere I bet."

"Now, Bob, you leave the poor girl alone. She's only just started. She's doin' fine. Don't wanna scare her off. Never have enough staff as it is." Pat turned to me, "Come and stand here beside me, love. As they come up, put a big scoop of mash on each plate and then they'll move on to me and Joan. We give 'em what meat they want and finally they get their veg and gravy from Betty at the end."

For the next half hour I stood there, with a long-handled metal scoop in one hand, holding onto a huge cauldron of mashed potato with the other, and dolloping some 150 servings onto some 150 plates. Almost every guy said something to me. Sometimes they were really friendly, sometimes probably taking the mickey. As I couldn't understand half they said, I just smiled and hoped for the best. It wasn't long before I had to switch to using my left hand, the right having become too painful

Worse was to come. Once all the men were served, Pat sent me to retrieve the first arrivals' empty plates. I knew I had to go out there, make an effort: smile, laugh, even try to parry their banter if I understood it, whatever was needed not to seem stuck up. But what with the wolf whistles and the frequent pats on my backside as I bent to retrieve the plates, by the time the factory siren went for work to restart, I had a thumping headache. There followed a great scraping of chairs on the slate floor as the men headed out. And I sighed with relief.

Pat sent me back into the canteen to wipe down the tables with disinfectant and sweep and mop the floor. It was some half hour later that I returned to the kitchen, just in time to see two women carrying great racks of clean cups over to be sterilised. I stepped in to help with what looked like a pretty dangerous operation. Together, we submerged the racks of cups in the vats of near boiling water and then hauled them, dripping, out again and onto massive draining boards.

Next came the job of drying the cups by hand and putting them away. I was exhausted, my head throbbed, my arm ached, and I watched in dismay as the women walked back and forth, back and forth, across the great kitchen carrying each cup in turn to be stacked ready for the following morning. Maybe if I hadn't been so tired I wouldn't have thought of it. But now I said, "Wouldn't it be easier if we let the racks drain a moment here and then carried them over there and dried the cups when we get there? It'd save an awful lot of walking." There was a long pause as the group thought about it and then Pat laughed.

"Hey, now that's not a bad idea! Come on, let's see if it works." And the women rallied round, made a space on the far side for the racks and helped lug them over. And thus I began to win acceptance among this team of older women standing around, chatting away and joking as they dried and restacked the crockery. While some of the gang cleaned the kitchen's industrial machines, I set to with dustpan and brush and then with mop and disinfectant to clean the floors.

At last it was time to clock out, find the bus stop and head home. I returned totally shattered and in ruddy awful pain. Exhausted physically because I was unused to heavy work but much more gutted mentally by the men's teasing and groping. Once I might have played up to them, given as good as I got. No more. Wanting only to collapse in a heap on my bed, I had instead to find the shops, buy bread and eggs, cereal and milk, jam and butter. I went to the post office, put in my father's birthday cheque, took out enough for my first month's rent and returned home.

Each day I had to force myself to get up, eat some cereals, catch the bus and go to work. Instead of the banter getting less as the week wore on, in my mind it seemed to grow worse.

One day on the way home I tried to stop off at the little park but soon a man came over and joined me on the bench. I jumped up and hurried away. Why sit next to me? What did he want?

By the end of the week, I'd had enough. I never signed up to be a waitress. I wouldn't have gone for the job if I'd known. I signed up to be a scullery maid. On Friday afternoon I collected my wage packet and left for good. I didn't say goodbye.

Making it on the outside was proving far harder than I'd expected. I'd become institutionalised without realising it. Apart from that short stay with Sue and another at home, I'd basically not done anything for myself going on for two years: no shopping, cooking or cleaning, let alone earning a living. Now I had to leave the house to buy food, find a chemist, go to the post office. My dread was that people would stare at me, judge me, find me wanting.

I took to wearing black: the black miniskirt and polo neck sweater from my birthday and the black suede lace-up boots that I'd worn on my London adventure with Hannah, plus the darkest of dark glasses. Thus, I hoped to become invisible. Surely no one would look at me dressed in black. I could pass like a phantom through the crowds of shoppers.

Unemployed, I had no wages coming in but, what with the money I'd saved over the years and now my father's birthday present, I calculated I could survive three months or more without a job. Not that survival was any longer part of my plan. The whole factory episode had reversed that, plunged me back into my gloom-filled quagmire. What was I good for? Nothing. Not even a scullery maid.

Gradually, as I lay on my bed day after day, all the colours once more drained from my world and again I saw only in shades of grey. Thoughts of suicide became my default. If there was no obvious reason to live, then clearly the answer was to die. Quit the whole hassle. Just stop eating. When next my food ran out, I didn't replenish it. I couldn't face going out. To begin with I felt pangs of hunger, but I eased these by drinking water. Days passed. I lay on my bed, waiting.

Then one afternoon my landlady called up the stairs, "Clare, you've some friends come to visit you!"

Sitting up, my head swam. Help! Who could be coming here looking for me? It turned out to be Jackie and Charles from The White House. They'd wheedled my address out of John, the social worker, and had come to pay a visit. I was still in my night clothes. I had been in the same clothes for a couple of weeks now. I invited them into my little kitchen.

"Hey! Have you got any coffee?" Charles asked as he opened an overhead cupboard—and then another. I pulled further back into the shadows, a rabbit trapped in the light.

Jackie turned, "But Clare! Where's your food? It's all empty! What's happened?"

I shrugged a shoulder and looked away. Malnutrition had made me too tired to try to explain. My head was still spinning from being upright. I couldn't think how to ward them off. Really it was no one's business but my own. These friends, who were they when you got down to it? Just people.

They didn't stay long and left worried. Later they told me that, when they got back to the White House, they told John what had happened, that they thought someone should visit me. He replied that, now I was 21, there was little they could do. If I wanted help, I'd have to ask for it.

A week later I had another visitor, a much more difficult one to ignore. As my letters dried up, my mother had driven over to check that I was okay. By the time she arrived I could barely stagger to the lavatory. I recognised at once her footsteps coming up the uncarpeted stairs. I decided to stay in bed.

Catching her breath at the top, Mum knocked on the closed bedroom door and called out, "Clare! Clare! It's me! Can I come in?" Heart hammering, I stayed still as a cornered mouse. I heard her head down the corridor and into the empty kitchen. What was she thinking? Maybe I'd gone out? Maybe got another job? Maybe... Hopefully she didn't go down that other road. I heard her return to my closed door and pause outside. "Clare, can I come in?"

I let out a faint "Yes." She opened the door. With the heavy, burgundy-coloured curtains drawn, it took her a while to adjust to the darkness. And then the smell must have hit her. The smell that went with unwashed clothes and unwashed bodies and windows all closed. She switched on the light. I sat up and she came and sat on the bed close beside me put a loving arm around me and held me close.

When I had finally told my parents I had discharged myself, Mum seemed quite pleased. She had hated what she considered that rundown, second-rate psychiatric hospital by the sea. Whereas we patients felt enabled by its malfunctioning organisation, she had feared it. Unlike us, she did not see it as a safe haven. She must have been reassured, even maybe hopeful, after the birthday celebration, with us all enjoying reminiscences of the past, recalling the good times of years gone by. If I had found myself a job and a bedsit all on my own, hopefully this would be a new start, the last year no more than a passing nightmare. But then the postman stopped dropping a weekly note through the letter box and she must have wondered what she should do. I was over twenty-one and jealous of my independence. Should she barge in like an overanxious mother or leave me, her daughter, to grow, to find my own way and, as Dad said, be ready to catch me if I fell.

"Sorry, Mum, I had a bad night. I was just trying to get some sleep. Why don't you pull back the curtains."

My mother got up. "How about I open the window too? You know it's pretty smelly in here, darling!" I had long since stopped noticing the smell. Returning to the bed she scrutinised me, my uncombed, tangled hair, my pinched face.

"How's the job going?"

I looked away. "I gave it up," I said in a voice devoid of expression. "It wasn't what the man said. I had to serve in the canteen too, not just clean the kitchen. I'd signed up to clean the kitchen and do the washing-up. After a week I left."

"Why didn't you write and tell us?"

"I didn't want you to worry."

Mum paused. "So what have you been doing since?"

"Nothing much. Lying here. Jackie and Charles called round a few days ago. But nothing much."

"Do you want to come back with me for a while and find a job nearer to home? Stay with us?"

I shook my head and mumbled, "No thanks, Mum. I'll manage."

She paused then rose from the bed. "How about I take some clothes and sheets home to wash? That way I can help." But I just shook my head again. She bent and kissed me lightly on the forehead. "Darling, you do know how much your father and I love you, don't you?"

I nodded and gave a meagre smile. "I love you too. I really do. It's me I hate." My eyes, gateway to my soul, must have looked empty, lost.

After my mother's visit, the world closed in around me. My bedsit was no longer a refuge. Darkness—black, suffocating—filled my head. I had to run. Right now. But where? *Stead! I need you!*

My whole body began to tremble as if I had DTs. As if some outer force had taken over and was shaking me. With quivering hands, severely weakened by 20 days without food, I struggled to pull off my nightdress; to climb into a black track suit; drag on a black coat. I found my keys and handbag; hid my eyes behind dark glasses and fled. I stepped aboard the first bus that came. "The sea," I muttered. "I want to go to the sea."

When the bus stopped, I was not too far from The Lady Chichester. Was it an instinct for life, making a final fling for my salvation, that led me, struggling, up the front steps and through the open door? Was this perhaps not so much a psychiatric hospital but a safe mooring in a storm?

Having arrived, the wild energy that had driven me vanished as if someone had pulled an electric plug from its socket. If a wooden bench hadn't been there to catch me, I would have fallen, a jumble of limbs, on the floor. Instead, I collapsed on the bench in the glass-enclosed porch. Even my teeth were chattering as if I'd just been dragged from a shipwrecked boat tossed in a raging sea.

I lost track of time, of reality. A nurse coming on duty found me and went in search of Dr Stead. He came: his face serious and concerned, his tall, lean frame slightly stooped. He sat on the bench beside me, put a sheltering arm around my shoulders and held me tight, trying to quiet my trembling.

"Life a bit too tough out there, eh?" He murmured in a quiet, sad voice. "I think we should give you an injection, Clare, just to see you through this bad patch."

Within the darkness, I registered that, for the first time, he had called me Clare.

He added in a more matter of fact voice, "Then I'll call an ambulance. The short-term ward of Brighton General can give you better care than we can offer here."

How strange that something which only a few months ago I would have fought tooth and nail, I now accepted without a whimper. Was it the days without food that had beaten down my resistance or was it the world?

The ambulance drove silently up the short semi-circle of drive and halted before The Lady Chichester's steps. The injection was already having an effect as they helped me up into the back and then eased me onto the stretcher inside. Stead leant over and wrapped the ambulance blanket more tightly around me. He patted my arm and said he'd see me soon. The vehicle drove silently away—more like a hearse than an ambulance.

14

Section 25

A LIFT TOOK US up to the hospital's acute psychiatric wing and there, after noting down my details, a nurse escorted me to the bathroom to change into a hospital gown and then led me to the 'quiet room'—in the bad old days known as a 'padded cell'. An ugly little room, its walls were indeed padded with a deep brown leatherette. On the floor was a mattress with sheets, pillow and blanket. I pushed the mattress to the edge of the room with my foot, lay down on it, curled up in a foetal position and turned my face to the wall.

The following morning, they led me into a large ward filled with two rows of white metal beds. I climbed into my designated berth, pulled the pillow close over my head and gently rock-rock-rocked myself in an effort to soothe the torment within. More tranquilisers. The nurse pulled away the pillow and told me firmly to take the pills and eat my lunch, in a tone that could have been aimed at a six-year-old. Vulnerable and dehydrated as I was, it worked. At least for the pills. Food was different. Starvation was now my chosen route to death. Pills hadn't worked. Gas hadn't worked. Exsanguination—as Hannah would have called it—hadn't worked. I took the pills, then lay still, staring blankly at the ceiling. White. Everything was white. The whole ward was white. The inside of my head was white—empty. No longer black but white.

Slowly, something crossed my field of vision. Emaciated, white-haired and dishevelled in a trailing hospital gown, the apparition stopped at my bed and fixed me with a fiery, witchlike stare. Very slowly she raised a skeletal arm and pointed a bony finger of accusation straight at me, mumbling in a monotone. Was she casting a spell? Cursing me? Inside my head, I laughed. *Am I not cursed enough? Am I not a curse simply by being alive?* For more than an hour the woman just stood, arm outstretched, catatonically condemning me. And the ward paid no attention. A nurse placed a tea tray on my bed table. I left it untouched and turned away from the accusing apparition. When I turned back both she and the tray had disappeared. Half an hour later Dr Stead arrived and sat down.

"Clare, Sister says you haven't eaten since you came here. Is that true?"

I nodded.

"Can you tell me why?"

"I'm not hungry. Not for food, life, anything."

"When did you last eat?"

I turned my head to stare down the long length of the ward. *He's going to ask 'why' next. Shall I just point down the ward? Ask what future is that?*

"I don't remember." I gave a slow shrug. *What does it matter? I'm not dead, am I?* "Maybe three weeks, something like that."

"Can you tell me about it?" He gently planted the question between us and then rested. The man had a stillness about him that was all accepting. One felt he could be trusted with anything. Maybe I, too, should trust him. After all he had been so very kind in holding me when I was in shock and calling me Clare, should I not reward him with something?

"I thought it was the best way to die. Most ways take effort and planning, cunning and courage. Not eating is a simple negative, totally passive; at least once one has learnt to ignore one's stomach's sharp-toothed pains."

Stead lent forward, an earnestness in his voice. "Clare, will you do something just for me? Will you please give up this starving idea? We've got enough problems to sort out without adding anorexia to the list." And he rose, picked up his driving gloves and bade me goodbye. "As you know, Clare, this is an acute psychiatric ward in a general hospital, just a holding ground before relocation. I'll try and have you transferred to The Villa. It's about 30 miles from here. I think you'll like it. It's a lot more modern than The Lady Chichester. It's meant mainly for young people with acute problems. You can still be my patient." And he gave a slight smile which penetrated to my heart and warmed it. Then he walked to the nurses' station, said he'd be in touch, flipped his gloves at them in farewell, and left.

It took Stead four days to arrange the transfer. Presumably the sister recorded in my ward notes that Clare Thompson had started eating. A desultory pecking but eating, nonetheless. On the fourth day they brought me my clothes, helped me dress, brushed my hair and did their best to make me look normal. *Ready for the next holding tank. Another clinic. Another bunch of people hoping to change me to someone else. Another group of people bound for failure.*

* * *

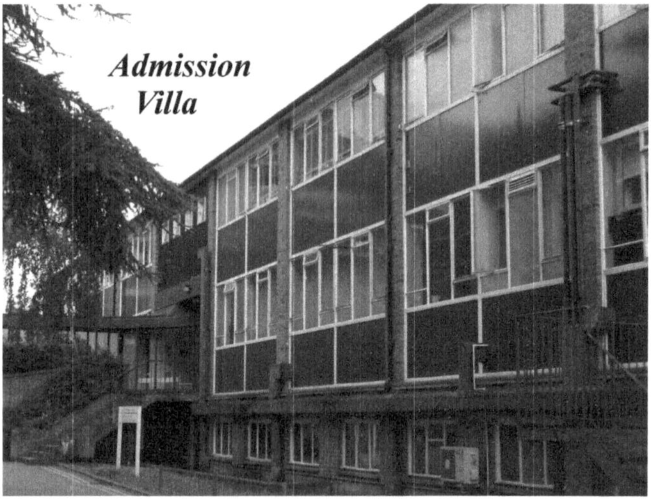

The Villa. [Credit: Joe Hughes]

The Villa, at the end of a tree-lined gravel drive, was a bright, modern, two-storey building with lots of glass—all unbreakable. Entering by some steps, reception was on the upper floor. The ground floor was divided in two: men one end, women the other. On the women's side on the left, a few small, individual rooms off a long corridor looked out over parkland. The last small room was called the Quiet Room. As in the Brighton General, it had a single mattress on the floor and a window onto the corridor so the nurses could see in, but the walls were painted white and thinly padded. Quite often patients themselves, fearing they were about to 'blow', would ask to go into the Quiet Room for twenty-four hours to calm down. Past it, at the end of the corridor, was a ten-bedded ward. The right-hand side of the corridor was lined with communal lavatories, bathrooms and storage cupboards.

Like all new patients, I was first placed in the small observation ward. Lying on top of my bed, exhausted, drained, I watched the other inmates apathetically through half-closed eyes. Right across from me, a little old lady sat stiffly upright in an armchair anxiously wringing her hands. She looked frightened. I was not altogether surprised as another patient, slight, young, with a mop of curly brown hair and blazing dark eyes was on a manic rampage.

"Hey all of you, look at me! I'm the greatest!" She jumped up, both fists punching the air. "I'm a genius! Did anyone tell you? I'm a genius! I'm studying medicine at Cambridge. Hey you!" She rushed at me. "What's your name? I'm Manda! I belong to Mensa! Come on, get off the bed! We've got to dance! Do you like the Beatles? I'm a great musician. I'll sing to you, and we can dance!" Then she rushed over to my neighbour. "Cathy, you gotta join us! Come on everyone! What's wrong with you? You all miserable? Up you get. We gotta dance. Let's dance down the corridor! Hey that'll be a laugh. Let's polka down the corridor. Up! Up! Up!" Unable to wait for a response, Manda set off alone polkaing to a tune in her head as she went, then, turning around, she sang all the way back into the ward.

At that moment Nurse Crawford, an elderly woman nearing retirement, called out "Manda! If you don't stop that racket we'll send you off to the Main Building! Here, I've got your Lithium[xxxii] for you. You love it, I know you do."

Manda danced over, grabbed the tiny cup of liquid, tossed it back like vodka and slapped the cup down on the nearest bedside locker. She then wiped her mouth on the back of her sleeve and danced away again.

I glanced over at Cathy, my neighbour, who smiled and gently shrugged one shoulder.

"Don't let Manda get to yer. She'll soon calm down. That Lithium works wonders."

Still weak, I lay on my bed, not speaking, gazing out through the large ward windows at the extensive hospital estate. The Main Building, St

Francis, stood just the other side of the parkland from The Villa. The place where they packed you away for good. At the start of the century, unmarried mothers, diagnosed as 'moral imbeciles', were locked up there for years along with their offspring. It was also the place that I'd told Stead I refused to go to.

On my second day, Mum arrived. I heard Sister introducing herself as they approached down the corridor. Sister Garrett was West Indian and walked with natural poise, head held high.[xxxiii] Dear Sister, her warm, kindly eyes no doubt shining with understanding at yet another distraught mother. Mum must surely have taken to her.

"I'm Clare's mother, Mrs Thompson. I've brought the clothes you asked for on the phone. Can I go in?"

"Well, Mrs Thompson, of course you can if you insist, but I think Clare needs a few more days to surface. Right now, she's not speaking. Why don't I take the case and then, once she settles in a bit more, you can visit her whenever you both agree."

Mum already knew that the psychiatrists preferred new admissions to be left in their care until they were responding to treatment, but she had come to see me. This time she must have decided to persevere, to put her needs first.

"That's very difficult for me, Sister. I need to see with my own eyes that she's okay. Then I'll leave. I promise."

"Alright, but just two minutes. And please don't feel upset. She's not responding right now but I'm sure she will after she's had a good rest. At least she's eating."

Mum followed Sister into the ward. She stood at the door searching for me then realised I was in the bed right beside her. I quickly closed my eyes, pretending to be asleep.

"Clare, it's me, darling. Just come to say hello." And she took my flaccid hand and gave it a squeeze and then bent over and kissed me on the forehead. Reluctantly I opened my eyes.

"Sister says she'll ring me when you are ready for visitors. I just wanted you to know that Dad and I are thinking of you and praying that you'll feel better soon. I think this looks like a good place for you." She scanned my face for a moment and for a moment I looked back.

"Right, I better go now, Sister's waiting to show me out."

There was a constant procession of patients being admitted and discharged. Manda was calmed and released. The old lady was given three ECTs and sent back to her retirement home.

On my first Wednesday at The Villa, a nurse escorted me upstairs to Dr Stead's consulting room and left me outside.

Sitting there alone, waiting, revived all my stomach-sickening fear of psychiatrists, even those I liked. And suddenly out of nowhere came a memory. It was to do with people being able to read my mind. I could see it vividly. Every year around Christmas we had a boisterous family party, some 20 people from three generations gathered together to play silly games, charades, maybe a treasure hunt or some Scottish dancing. Our host, Uncle Bill,[xxxiv] was a charismatic man, a doctor, with fine features and very perceptive grey eyes. Once John had told me to be wary of him. He said Uncle Bill could read my mind.

From that moment on, I had refused to speak to the man, indeed did everything I could to avoid him altogether until just after I left school. I was seventeen and we were sitting on the floor in a circle playing my father's favourite, crazily competitive game called La-di-da, when I found myself next to Bill. And he cheated. Pretending to be outraged, I called out teasingly that he was a rotten cheat. Everyone laughed and then he teased me back and I relaxed and realised he could be very charming.

As we went to say goodbye, I overheard Bill saying to my mother. "Ro, congratulations! That daughter of yours has grown up so much since last year. Definitely more entertaining!" Later, when I was nursing, I discovered my Uncle Bill had helped to pioneer the EEG or electroencephalogram machine that measured brainwaves; hence John's mind-reading story. He even invited me over to the National Hospital, Queen Square, where he was in charge, to see the huge mainframe that had performed one of the world's first EEGs. Could it be that that ancient machine that read brainwaves was the hidden origin for my present fear?

A few minutes later Dr Stead arrived, startling me from my reverie. "Ah Miss Thompson, good afternoon. How are you settling in?" I was back to being Miss Thompson.

"Okay," I said, my voice stiff and wary.

"What were you thinking about so deeply that I made you jump?"

"Nothing. Childhood. Christmas."

"Was it happy?"

I smiled tentatively. "Yes, very! Lots of us. All ages. Three families of cousins and my mother's spinster aunts."

"And how are you feeling now?"

"Now? Dead. Numb. Nothing."

"I've been remembering how I found you shaking in the porch at The Lady Chichester and wondering what we can do to help. Obviously, I can't swear that this time it will work but I've come to the conclusion we should give ECT one more try."

I stared at him with a stunned sense of betrayal—and by Stead.

"Of course," he continued, "now you're twenty-one, we'll need your consent. If you agree, you just need to sign here." Dr Stead eased a form across the 'sanity' table and held out his fountain pen.

No! Electro-convulsive therapy, that softly hissing euphemism. Never again! My brain won't survive. Sixteen ECTs and all that deep narcosis too, to say nothing of 16 general anaesthetics. My brain'll shrivel up and die.

I still believed life was not worth living. Nevertheless, I refused point blank to sign away what was left of my brain.

"Never!" I whispered.

Dr Stead spoke quietly, compassion mingling with determination in his tired voice. "I'm sorry Miss Thompson, but if you don't sign this, I'm afraid we'll have to Section you, and you know what that means."

I hadn't been shuffled around the psychiatric circuit for well over a year without learning what it meant to be Sectioned.

They no longer certified us insane. That wasn't 'nice'. Instead, they Sectioned us under Part IV, Section 25 of the Mental Health Act, 1959. It came to the same thing, of course. Just two doctors' signatures and all our rights evaporated, leaving us at the mercy of those same doctors to do what they liked. Murderers had better protection.

Sectioned, I would, by law, have to comply with whatever treatment my doctors prescribed. Alternatively, if I signed Stead's form, it would allow them to administer 10 more ECTs in the hope of propelling my mind out of suicidal darkness. It hadn't worked before. It had played havoc with my intellect. If they wanted what remained of my brain cells they'd have to fight me for them. I refused to sign.

The two of us sat on in silence, the untouched consent form lying, oppressive, between us. Finally, Dr Stead glanced at his watch and snapped the cap back on his fountain pen.

"I think you're making a mistake. I don't want to do it, but I'm afraid now we'll have to Section you. You'll receive a letter shortly."

As he left the room, I remained motionless. There seemed little point in moving.

Eventually a nurse appeared bearing a letter in a long manila envelope.

MENTAL HEALTH LEAFLET NO 1

Dear Miss Thompson,

You have been admitted to this hospital for treatment under Part IV of the Mental Health Act, 1959. Dr Stead is in charge of your treatment here and is responsible for deciding when you may leave the hospital. You have the right under the Act to apply to the Mental Health Tribunal... If you wish to do so you must do so on a special form which you can obtain by writing to the Tribunal...

In 1959 mental *illness* had been sanitised, becoming mental *health*. A wry smile flickered across my face. With some tens of thousands of people held under Section 25 in British psychiatric institutions. I wondered how many of society's untouchables—the manic, the psychotic, the depressed and the non-conforming—had the self-confidence, let alone the mental clarity to appeal. I decided instead to run away.

15

Escape Artist

SICK WITH ANXIETY, I hovered until the convoy of ECT patients had formed. A nurse sailed at their head but there was no battleship to bring up the rear. Did they think we were already too crushed to rebel? Joining last, I waited until I reached the foot of the staircase which led upwards towards freedom. I bent swiftly and slipped off my clumsy Dr Scholl's then darted, silent and barefoot, up the stairs.

Tiptoeing past reception, I sped down the outside steps, my white hospital gown flapping, wraith-like behind me. Along the gravelled drive, fear numbed my feet. Fear gave me speed, burst in my lungs and hammered inside my skull. On and on I ran. Ahead lay a coppice. If only I could reach its shelter.

But now I heard footsteps behind me; heavy shoes crunching on the gravel, heavy breathing carrying with it the menace of capture. I plunged blindly into the wood. Mud squelched between my toes. Brambles caught at my gown and scratched my naked flesh. Fear gave me strength to break free. But then a root reached out and tripped me up. I fell, sprawling, into the mud.

There I lay still, all fire quenched. A shadow crossed my closed eyelids. A man in a white coat knelt to lift me in his arms. Slowly, panting from his exertions, he carried me out of the woods, murmuring reassurances as if I was a frightened kitten—or a young woman, unhinged. Through my mind flitted an image of my father. When I was little, after a long car journey, sometimes I used to pretend to be asleep just to have him pick me up in his warm arms and carry me indoors

Later, the same nurse who had picked me up drew the thorns one by one from my bruised and battered feet. But I was no longer there. From high above the bed, I looked down impassively on the male nurse and the wounded girl. *Compassion, too, is one of their weapons. They use caring to break down our resistance, to lure us back from our difference into the fold of 'normality'.*

*　　　*　　　*

Two days later Nurse Crawford was detailed to deliver me personally to the ECT treatment centre. Recipients were confined to bed without breakfast, then at 9 a.m., dressed in hospital gowns, they were led single-file down the long, lower corridor towards the men's end of the building. Both sexes were herded into a waiting room with one small window set high up near the ceiling. On that first treatment day, I shared a wooden bench with a scraggly, middle-aged stranger. Squashed close beside him, I could physically sense his fear.

"Don't be afraid," I murmured. "It only makes it worse."

"Can't help it. Had it before. Back in the fifties." Briefly the man's body shuddered against mine. "They used to strap you down then. Tie you to the table and ram a gag between your teeth. So's you didn't bite your tongue when you had the fit, like. They did it cold."

"It's different now. Truly. They anaesthetise you. It doesn't hurt. In fact, I quite like the feeling. It's like floating down a warm silken tunnel into a dream." I turned to our companions. "Shall we ask if he can go first?" In that small room, heavy with anxiety, the waiting was the worst. The dread of not knowing how you would be when you came round: mildly confused, splitting headache, verging on gaga? Typical of the solidarity of patients, everyone agreed. It was then just a matter of persuading the nurse to ask the anaesthetist to change the patient order.

Later that afternoon, Cathy said, "Why don't yer come and sit over in the window? It's good over there."

So I went with Cathy to sit by the ward's large, unbreakable windows that looked across broad meadowland towards the South Downs. Cathy was as tall as me—and almost as thin. She had short mousy hair and a wistful face from which arrestingly pale blue eyes looked mournfully out onto the world.

"Are yer from near 'ere?"

"Yes, not far. I was in The Lady Chichester for a while, down on the coast. Discharged myself on my 21st birthday." I paused. "But I couldn't make it out there. So now I'm here."

"It's not bad 'ere, not really. I've seen worse. They brought me in two weeks ago. Most of the staff are okay. The ward doctor, Dr Pirrie, is real nice. Dr Stead visits sometimes." She fell silent for a long moment. "Don't know 'bout you but they've labelled me schizophrenic. Say I hallucinate. It's because sometimes I 'ear voices." The last comment was followed by a swift glance to see my reaction.

I didn't react at all. They were all just labels. At the time, the US diagnosed most patients as schizophrenic whilst the British catch-all category was 'depressive'. Didn't seem to make much odds. In fact, each patient's problems were a unique perplexity.

Soon Cathy and I discovered that we were almost identical in age, both 21, but from very different backgrounds and admitted for very different reasons. Cathy was already married with five children. Yes, five by the age of 21.

As the days passed, we became close friends. Some days Cathy's voices were so overpowering she couldn't concentrate enough to carry on a conversation, eat a meal, drink a cup of coffee. Sometimes those voices shouted in her head telling her she was wicked, the Devil incarnate. Then she'd bash her head against a wall trying to shut those voices up—until a member of staff came to give her an injection and help her into bed. But on other days, when her voices were less strident, Cathy shared childhood memories with me.

"My dad was crazy. I mean real, ravin' mad, crazy. The neighbours said he was a true lunatic. Come the full moon he'd beat up our mum something vicious plus whichever of us kids as took his fancy. We tried to protect me mum, but we were scared too. There was five of us, three boys, me sister Jan, and me. I was the youngest. When Dad was nuts and the boys young he sometimes forced 'em to go to school wearin' gumboots and girls' dresses."

Another time, over lunch, Cathy said, "Our mum was the breadwinner. Dad never kept a job more than a few weeks before he got in a fight. He was always drinkin'. Mum went out cleanin'—shops mainly. One day, walkin' home, she saw this grandfather clock in a junk shop. It was all in warm, polished woods, and she fell in love with it. Not like me mum at all. Usually dead practical, careful with money an' all. Mind you, she had to be."

Cathy paused, a faraway look in her pale blue eyes. She went on. "Still, she got the shop to put that clock on one side. She went in each week on pay day and paid it off, bit by little bit. Took her over two years. Finally, she'd paid every last penny and she and the boys carried it home. Triumphant, they were!" Cathy smiled at the memory. "She looked *so* happy. Don't think I ever saw her look happier. Until that night, when the rotten bastard took a hammer to it. Said she shouldn't ought to have bought it. Smashed it to matchsticks. Nothing left. It wasn't so long after that that me voices came visiting."

A week later I finally received my day clothes and, thus liberated, set out to explore the rest of the building. As I passed one of the single rooms, I heard a baby crying and peered in. Juliet, a young woman in her mid-twenties with a shock of black hair to match that of her tiny child, was standing at the window. They'd been brought in as an emergency after Juliet developed postnatal depression. More recently, she and her little boy had been moved out of the admissions ward and into a single room. Now I noticed the window stood wide open. It was cold outside, and the distressed mother had put her new-born babe, stark naked, on the stone windowsill while she rubbed him vigorously with some sort of oil.

I turned on my heels and hurried back to the nurses' station.

"Sister, I think Juliet and the baby need you. She's got him lying out on the windowsill. He's got no clothes on."

Sister rose gracefully, "Thank you, Clare. That's good you came and told me." And she walked silently down the corridor in her soft-soled shoes.

Taking the stairs, I found my way to the large, upstairs common room where male and female patients, at least those allowed day clothes, could meet. Cathy was already there and I went to join her on the long sofa; though

I was careful not to sit too close. I had noted early on that many patients needed extra personal space, didn't like people sitting too near them.

Cathy was having a good day. We started chatting. "Did I ever tell you how I got married? Why I got married?" I shook my head.

"I just couldn't stand me dad one more day. I reckon if I'd stayed a moment longer I'd have taken an axe to him and butchered him. Blood splattered all over the walls! I was sixteen. Ran away with Johnny, didn' I. He was eighteen and had a good job as a brickie. Me mum signed for the marriage. She knew as why I'd run off. Guess we thought we were in love." She smiled. "We set up house and I started having babies. Got a council flat. In the end it turned out Johnny was as bad as me old man. Drank too much, then turned mean. They say that about the daughters of alcoholics. That we often marry alcoholics ourselves. Maybe it's 'cos that's what we're used to? Better the devil yer know?" Cathy took a weary breath. "As the family grew we got a proper council house. A nice one an' all. I was expectin' our fifth when Johnny kicked me in the belly, upped sticks an' left." Cathy paused to gaze out of the window.

Then she looked over at me, her eyes pleading for understanding. "I couldna' do it, Clare, I couldna'. Not without Johnny to help me, I couldn't cope. Not after little Susie was born. I adored those kids. Still do. They were everythin' to me. Then I started hearin' voices. Telling me crazy things to do to 'em. Sometimes I'd beat me head against the wall to try and shut them voices up. I got a family allowance but I couldn't even work out how to shop or cook."

"Oh Cathy, that's awful! You poor thing! But don't blame yourself. I'm quite sure there's hardly anyone could cope with all that!"

"It was a neighbour as reported me to social services. They sent a social worker round to check the house. Didn't give me no warning, nothin'. Well of course it was a tip, wasn't it! Hadn't cleaned it for weeks. There were all these dirty nappies lyin' around. I couldn't handle it, Clare. I was desperate." Cathy fished out a handkerchief to blow her nose.

"Then they came and took all the kids away. Put them in care and I haven't even been allowed access. It was then I tried to kill meself. What was the point of livin' without them? My children! I loved them, Clare. I love 'em now. More than anything in the world. They're mine. All I've got."

And Cathy buried her head in her hands and wept. Space or not, I moved close and put my arm around her and rocked her and held her tight.

Stead sent me off for yet another IQ test. The next time I saw him I asked, "Have you had my results back yet?"

"Yes. You got 135. I was slightly surprised it wasn't higher."

"It was. The last time I took one maybe two years ago, it was 20 points higher. So I guess all that ECT and deep narcosis not only wiped out my memory but killed off my intelligence too."

Eventually I graduated to my own room. As the days passed and the ECTs accumulated, I became more and more restless. I had to get out. Not run away exactly, just out. Out into the countryside and the fresh air. Away from people. People! I needed solitude. Silence. I knew I should ask. But what if the answer was no?

So, I asked no one. I chose a Saturday morning for my country walk as there was no ECT that day, no one keeping close tabs on me. Also, several patients would be going home for the weekend. I waited near the stairs for a family group to set out and simply tagged along behind them and walked out through the front door.

Autumn was approaching. I decided to take the old, sunken lane I remembered from childhood that bordered the far side of the vast hospital grounds. I'd follow it down to a little stream that we'd delighted in as children, where slender silver birches rose from the banks, their leaves softly rustling. Wearing Wellington boots, we all three had paddled and splashed in a shallow ford and built dams out of stones.

Once outside the grounds, I felt my spirits rise. It was a couple of miles to the start of the lane and then, as its ancient banks rose high beside me, I began to dance. A dance of freedom? I laughed and twirled and sang Scott McKenzie's latest hit about going to San Francisco wearing flowers in your hair. I paused to pluck white blossoms from the hedgerows and twist them in amongst my wavy locks, for recently I'd let my hair grow long.

I hadn't felt so good for weeks, maybe years. Maybe this was it. Maybe at last the dark clouds were rolling back forever! Then, even as I thought it, I heard a car approaching down the narrow lane behind me. I stepped close into the bank to let it pass. Too late I saw it was a police car. The lone driver stopped and rolled down his window. "Hey love, is your name Clare?"

I stared at him, not saying a word. I saw his eyes flick up to my hair and I remembered the flowers. *Do I look mad?* I wondered. I put a tentative hand up to remove them then decided not to. I liked them there. Somehow, they showed I belonged to something, a sort of wayward member of the hippy movement, in love with peace and brotherhood.

Reluctantly I gave a slight nod.

"We've been looking for you, you know. Hop in and I'll give you a lift back to The Villa. They rang us, worried about you."

I hesitated and then, seeing no escape, climbed grudgingly in beside him and turned my head away. Minutes before, I'd been so crammed full of joy. I'd been like a skirling bagpipe and now I was more like a punctured goatskin from which all joy had seeped away.

The policeman started up the car, drove to the end of the sunken lane to get better reception and pulled over next to the stream. He picked up the dashboard walkie-talkie and called Police Headquarters.

"I've found the girl. She's okay. I'm driving her back now. Over."

Above the speaker's crackles, I heard the man at the other end replying, "Go careful with her, Jim. Remember she's Sectioned. They say she's a high suicide risk. Over."

"Yes, thanks Ken. I know. She's okay. Over and out." And the young policeman quickly switched off his receiver. "Don't you pay no attention to that, love. It's just stuff we need to write in reports and things."

For a while we drove in silence then Jim turned towards me. "What's it like in there? Awful?" He wasn't that much older than me.

I paused, my brain still swimming with the defeat of it all. "No," I said, my voice quavering distantly through the fog inside my head. "Not awful. They give you shock treatments. That mushes up your brains, but I wasn't running away. I just had to get out. One feels so impotent. Like a prisoner. A prisoner of the Freudian thought police."

Arriving, Jim got out and opened the door for me, a small courtesy or kindness that raised my wilted spirits. He walked up the steps with me and waited in the lobby while the receptionist phoned down for Sister Garrett.

"So Clare, welcome back! We were worried when we couldn't find you. Couldn't you have told us you wanted to go out?"

"I was afraid you'd say no. I had to get out!" I heard myself sounding like a petulant teenager.

Sister Garrett turned to the policeman. "Thank you very much, Officer. We can take care of her now."

Jim turned and smiled at me. "You look after yourself, love. I'm sure you'll be let out soon."

Two days later Dr Stead called for me. He opened the door and ushered me into his office.

"So how are you feeling?"

I lifted my eyes slowly to his face, stared at him for a second and then slid my gaze away. Since my return in the police car, the black clouds had come rolling in.

Dr Stead considered me for a moment. Did he, too, note the resurgence of that leaden despair? "I've been wondering, Miss Thompson. Do you remember your comment when we very first met? At the hospital? That you said you'd never go to St Francis, the Main Building, here? Do you remember that? Have you ever thought that maybe right now you're trying to force me to send you there, subconsciously you understand? You shake your head, but it may be that this is the real reason why you refuse to co-operate. Maybe you really want us to punish you; lock you up in the 'lunatic asylum' next door; throw you on the muckheap where you feel you belong and throw the key away. Think about it. Maybe that is what you really want. The punishment you think you deserve. For some sin you believe you've committed? The pain that will assuage the guilt? The crown of thorns? The martyrdom. Does that idea ring bells with you?"

I sat, immobile and expressionless.

"As I say, think about it. We'll see how you manage over the next few weeks. As you know, The Villa is only meant for short-term, two or three-month, acute psychiatric cases. It's not intended for chronic clinical depression."

Back in my room I collected writing paper and ballpoint pen and wrote:

Dear Doctor Stead

In all the months we've known each other I believe I have never asked you for anything before. But I'm asking you now. Please, please don't ever send me to the Main Building. I won't die there. I'll go out of my mind. I know I will.

Yours sincerely
Clare Thompson

In fact, both Cathy and I were pushing the boundaries of the Villa's stipulated short-term acute psychiatric care, and neither was getting any better. We hung out together most days, usually in the upstairs communal day room. Sometimes Joe, a very shy young man would join us from the men's ward. He, too, had attempted suicide. His father was a bit like Cathy's, except he wasn't an alcoholic, he was worse: a cold-blooded psychopath. He thought Joe was a wimp and regularly beat him, to toughen him up you understand!

One day Joe shared with us a story that he said he'd never shared before.

"As a kid I only had one real friend. I know it sounds daft but it was a pet duck." We smiled encouragingly at him as he paused. "Mum persuaded Dad to allow me to keep her. I called her Angel, 'cos she was my Angel. She followed me everywhere. When I walked to the front gate to go to school, Angel came along right beside me. When I came back, Angel was waiting there ready to welcome me home with outspread wings.

He hesitated, stared at the floor just in front of his feet, bit at the quick of one, well-gnawed nail, composed himself, and went on. "Then one day when I was ten, I came home from school and Angel wasn't there. That night we had roast duck for supper." Joe's voice trembled and his eyes welled up with tears. "He made me eat her," he whispered.

Cathy and I sat in shocked silence staring at him. What could you say to a story like that? Maybe it was time I dropped my scorn for those who heaped blame on parents for their children's mental sickness? Maybe it was me that was the odd one out?

16

London Revisited

WINTER HAD ARRIVED early and ever since my ramble down the country lane my street clothes had been locked away and I had been shut up indoors. I was going stir-crazy. That black madness was again welling up inside me. I had to break free!

I had been planning my escape for weeks. There was really little else to do. I'd told Mum that I no longer wanted my shabby blue dressing gown. Instead, could she please bring in my thick, black poncho, the one the Mexican Military attaché had presented to Dad? It would make a change, less like a hospital uniform. I also asked for my black, baby-doll nightdress. I didn't mention that I thought it could pass as a mini-dress, though painfully thin for a winter's day.

The following Saturday I ate a big breakfast then dressed in the diaphanous mini nightdress and the black poncho and slid my feet into my Dr Scholl sandals. I was going to take the train to London. To the Embankment to be precise, for I was going to become a tramp, and I knew that's where tramps slept, on the benches along the Embankment beside the River Thames.

I collected together my wash things, a spare pair of knickers and my precious powder compact in which, months ago, I'd hidden a blank cheque and razor blade ready for a rainy day and packed them into a drawstring bag. Again, I tagged on behind patients going out through the front door and walked briskly to the bus stop just around the corner from the hospital's main entrance. Being on home territory, with my parents' house only five miles away, I knew the bus routes and the railway station and where I could draw money with my cheque. Once I got to London, I'd use the money to buy jeans and socks, a thick sweater and newspapers to wrap myself in at night. Tramps, I knew, always had newspapers to keep themselves warm and the consensus amongst The Chich's inmates, several of whom had lived on the streets, was that *The Times* afforded the best insulation.

There was no one at the bus stop, which at first was a relief as I had been frightened an off-duty nurse might recognise me. But soon I realised there was no one there because a bus must have just left. I was getting colder by the minute. My bare toes were already numb and my knees felt like balls of blue ice. I pulled the rough poncho closer round me so at least my upper body was warm. By the time the bus arrived my teeth were chattering, and I was so cold I felt ill. Sheer pig-headedness kept me going.

The bank proved no trouble at all. To be on the safe side, I decided to take out the large sum of ten pounds in one-pound notes, enough to buy all I needed and more. (That's around £180 in today's money.) From the bank it was but a short walk to the railway station where I defrosted in the waiting room until the next train came in. Sitting at the window watching the grey, gaunt trees flash by, I remembered nostalgically the last time I'd gone to London, with Hannah. We still kept in touch by letter, but I felt really uncomfortable when visiting her and her partner. The latest news was that they were expecting a baby. Hannah and I were slipping apart.

Once in London, I headed first for a news stand and bought four copies of *The Times*. Then I went into the chemist next door to buy Codeine. I'd forgotten just how painful my arm was without the DF118, but those came only on prescription. Now I'd need some bottled water to go with them. Finally, I searched out a charity shop near the station and bought a stout pair of jeans, thick socks, two warm sweaters, a scarf and some tough-looking boots and put them all on in the changing room. I asked for a carrier bag and added the newspapers, my drawstring bag and my Dr Scholls to it. Life began to look a bit brighter.

Three stops on the Tube brought me to Embankment Station and there, in front of me, lay the Thames. I hurried towards it, eager to embrace my new home. Then stopped abruptly. The benches were there alright, but some misanthropic busy-body had divided them all up with wrought-iron arm rests so the homeless couldn't stretch out. In anger I plonked myself down, put the carrier bag on the bench beside me and reviewed the situation. I dredged through what was left of my mind, trying to remember what else I knew about living on London's streets. Sometimes people slept under railway bridges, but I had no idea where to find one. Doorways? There were always doorways. I'd better try to find a doorway before it got dark. But what if they're all taken? What if there's a rota for the best doorways, like there's one for London's best busking pitches? Still, doorways it would have to be.

Gathering up the bag, I crossed the Embankment once more and retreated inland from the river. Wandering further into the darker part of town, I eventually found a likely piece of property: a passage leading into an office block. Maybe that would do? Protected from the wind and rain. Unlikely to be spotted in the dark. Presumably there was no one in the office block at this hour so I'd not be in anyone's way. Going into the far corner, I took one copy of *The Times*, folded it in half, dropped it on the ground and eased myself down onto it. Then I leaned back against the cold wall. I fished out another newspaper and wrapped it clumsily around my legs. The final two papers were destined for my shoulders and chest. With some difficulty I enveloped myself in these with the poncho to keep them in place. But what happens if the wind gets up? It'll blow the paper right off my legs. Why did I never study street dwellers more carefully? Now one of them, I felt that 'tramp' or vagabond was perhaps too derogatory for these ingenious people, these survival experts. It was all much more complicated than I'd imagined.

I tried to sleep. But not for long. Soon I was woken by a shoe gently prodding at my leg. "Hey! You can't sleep there. The police'll move you on in no time. I'd go that-a-way," and the man pointed down a narrow street lined with tenement buildings. "Thank you," I said, my voice pale with exhaustion.

Again, I folded my papers and moved on. Again, I found a doorway and tried to settle but half an hour later a bag lady came along. Considerably the worse for wear, the old woman swayed over my feet. "What d'yer think you're doing mucking up our neighbourhood! You get yer dirty carcass out of my sight or I'll call the police!" So much for the camaraderie of the streets.

Time trickled by. The pain in my arm was getting worse. Over recent months, protected by DF118, I'd barely thought about my arm. I got out the water bottle and swigged down two more Codeine. It would need at least half an hour before they worked. Meanwhile my morale was tumbling as I slunk into yet another doorway, but I couldn't sleep. I was too scared. One hour, two hours? A rough-looking man spotted me.

"Can't stay there, ducks, the cops'll be along soon."

"Where should I go then?" Even to my ears I sounded pathetic, almost tearful.

Slowly I collected up my crumpled papers, picked myself up, and moved out onto the street.

I don't know how long I walked. The sounds of the city grew softer. The odd police siren made me pull in close to the wall. The streets became narrower and I colder. The heat of my defiance faltered. Exhausted, I came to a wider thoroughfare with a bus shelter. I rested on the bench. A late-night double-decker pulled up, its golden lights warmly beckoning me inside. VICTORIA was emblazoned across the front. Victoria, the railway station that led back home. It was too much to resist. I decided to give up.

I got in, paid the fare and sat down near the front. At Victoria Station I struggled into the near-empty concourse and collapsed at the foot of one of the tall pillars. Inside, my head felt weird and empty. It was many hours since I'd had any medicine apart from the Codeine or, for that matter, anything to eat. All I wanted to do now was sleep.

It was there, at the foot of the pillar that a bobby bent down and gave me a shake.

"Hey! Yer can't sleep here, you know. Where're you from?"

I looked at him—and decided not to say.

"Up yer get. We'll go to the office and then you can tell us." Linking his arm firmly under my armpit he pulled me to my feet. A few minutes later I found myself inside the Victoria Station transport police office sitting in an old-fashioned wooden armchair at the far side of a large wooden desk.

"So can you tell us what your name is, love?"

"Clare,"

"Clare what?"

"Clare Thompson." Then I lowered my voice. "You're looking for me."

"What's that?"

"You're probably looking for me," I repeated, louder this time.

"Really. So why's that then?"

"I'm on the run."

"On the run! From where?"

"The Villa psychiatric clinic."

"So where's that?" But I'd changed my mind. I refused to say any more. "Hang on, I'll just check this out." The policeman picked up his phone and dialled. After a long, slightly muffled conversation he hung up and turned to me. "So, seems you're right. Now we've got to work out how to get you back."

In the end it was my father who collected me from Haywards Heath station. "Hello poppet!" It always made me feel warm and wistful when he used his childhood name for me. "Where shall I take you? You can come home to us, or I can take you back to the Villa."

"To the Villa please." A silence came between us.

"You know Clare, your mother and I never wanted you to go to this place. But we didn't know what else to do. Even worse would be if you killed yourself. We felt that here they can protect you until you get better."

"It's okay, Dad. I understand. I told you before, in your place I'd probably do the same."

A few days later, on 7th January 1968, I received a letter from my father.

My Darling,

I wonder whether in future, when you feel you must get away from everyone, I could drive you somewhere where you could get out and go for a long walk on your own—I wouldn't talk to you at any time—unless you wanted me to.

My love
Daddy

On my return to the Villa, I withdrew one step further into myself. Dr Stead was seeing me twice a week in the hope that, somehow, they would make a breakthrough; discover the buried source of all this darkness, self-hatred and fear. For I was becoming more and more afraid. Afraid of everything: of people, of treatment, of Dr Stead. I refused to speak during our sessions though I did write him letters, sometimes 10 and 15 pages long. I had to be alone.

Alone because I felt so responsible. I'd always found it easy to empathise with people, put myself in their shoes and my time as a nurse had turned me into a good listener. Even now, patients sought me out to unburden themselves—and I felt caught in an ever-tightening web of liability. What if they were to kill themselves? It would be all my fault. I had to be alone.

One day I was walking along the downstairs corridor when I saw the hospital superintendent and a small group of teenage secondary school students heading towards me. I searched frantically for somewhere to hide. But there was nowhere. So I turned my back on them and, pressing my face into the wall, I cupped my hands around the sides of my head until they had passed, like a small child thinking that if it couldn't see it couldn't be seen.

As they went by, I heard the superintendent say. "That's Clare. She's suffering from severe depression."

Maybe this was it. Maybe I was now going truly mad?

An hour later I went to Sister Garrett and asked, for the first time, to go into the Quiet Room. I had never done anything like that before but now I felt as if, at any moment, I would explode like a supernova and fall deeper still into my black hole. Dressed only in my pyjamas and dark glasses, I lay down on the mattress, curled myself into a ball and didn't move. Except for visits to the lavatory, I lay still for three days. I didn't speak. I didn't eat and I hardly drank at all. But, after three days of complete quiet, I slowly emerged from my dark confusion and began to function normally again, to wish to see Cathy, to talk to Dr Stead. The padded cell, the isolation, had eased my stressed-out soul.

17

The Truth

THE PSYCHIATRIST IN charge of the women's ward, Dr Pirrie, was a relaxed, friendly man with an alternative attitude to mental illness. He believed as much in promoting the healthy side of his patients as in burrowing into their shortcomings. One day he came up beside me in the corridor. "Are you going to the talk on contraception? It's in about ten minutes. You should go, you know." And he laughed. "You might need it one day. How about we go together?"

I reckoned, as a nurse, I knew all there was to know on the subject, but I liked Dr Pirrie and to go to anything with him would not only be a pleasure but also revolutionary in the scenario of strict doctor/patient relationships. Besides, it would relieve the tedium.

The common room was already crowded when we arrived. The chief interest centred around the new contraceptive pill. When it was first introduced by the British National Health Service in 1961, doctors were only allowed to prescribe it to married women. It wasn't until 1967 that it was to become universally available. So, for most of the patients, young and old, it was still a bit of a mystery.

After the talk, Dr Pirrie and I left together and, on the way back downstairs, he put a friendly arm around my shoulders. "You know, Clare, you're okay. You shouldn't be so down on yourself. You're going to be okay, I know you are." Then he patted me on the back and walked off, leaving me standing at the foot of the stairs, non-plussed. No psychiatrist in all those months had ever said that I was okay!

It took another couple of weeks of ground-floor living before Cathy and I finally graduated together to neighbouring rooms upstairs.

On the second floor we had much more freedom. I begged Dr Pirrie to allow me to have a gramophone in my room so I could listen to music. He agreed. Dad came over the following Saturday with my old gramophone and a small box of vinyl LPs. We sat in the visitors' area of the entry hall and chatted for a while but, as always, I sensed my father's discomfort. For a former army officer there was something very gentle about him. He loved ballet and watercolour painting, horse riding and theatre. He was a faithful but never 'pushy' Christian. He loved me, his daughter dearly, I knew that, but he didn't really do 'chat'. Serious debate with John on some topical subject clearly gave him great pleasure—but chat?

"You do know, Clare, that your mother and I would do anything in our power to make you happy again. But we simply don't know how."

That, for my father, was quite a speech and I gave him a quick hug. "Thanks for bringing the records." I said as I stood up and, picking up my gramophone, headed to my room. I felt slightly smug: the only person in the Villa with their own music centre.

A few days later I received a letter from my father. He, like me, was better at communicating by the written rather than the spoken word.

Clare Darling,

... against a background of love, all I want to do is to offer bridges in case you should want to cross—I do not touch or kiss you because I believe that you believe that you would not like it. But in case you should ever want a shoulder to cry on, which might not be a bad idea, mine is always available—I don't think I have put this very well but I have so much more belief in you than you have yourself—Whatever you may think, you have the talents and ability to do so much to make this old world a better place.

With love
Daddy

It was after we moved up to the second floor that Cathy and I were prescribed a new 'wonder' drug. By the mid-sixties, Mandrax had ousted barbiturates as the psychiatrists' sleeping potion of choice—not only had barbiturates proved addictive but there was no antidote to an overdose. We were both prescribed 300mg of the drug each night. Mentioning this to one of her brothers, Cathy learned that Mandrax, or Mandies, had recently become one of his favourite recreational drugs. But it was we who discovered the trick of chewing them to enhance their effect. In those susceptible, Mandrax was said to, 'induce relaxation, remove sexual inhibitions and increase feelings of happiness and calm'.

Every evening after supper, Cathy and I would wait for the night staff to come round with the sedatives. We'd take our Mandrax, pretend to swallow them and wait for the staff to leave. Then we'd sit together on the floor of my room, the gramophone between us, chew our pills—and wait for the high.

With the sound turned right down, we played our way through my collection of records, mainly Joan Baez and Bob Dylan but also close harmony specialists like Simon and Garfunkel. The words of their recently released *Sound of Silence* resonated deep inside my alienated heart. Then there were The Seekers with their *Carnival is Over* and Peter, Paul and Mary's *500 Miles*. I realise now that it was in my bedroom at the Villa, sitting cross-legged on the floor, listening to those songs of protest, that the foundations of my life philosophy were laid. Dylan's anti-war song, *Blowin in the Wind*, and Baez' *Prison Trilogy*, songs for justice and peace became my benchmark for how human beings should behave towards one another. Spaced out and relaxed, I found solace in those soul-sad songs. They harmonised with the desolation that was, once more, painting dark shadows on the inside of my mind and they put me in touch with emotions I'd suppressed for so long that I could no longer evoke them at will.

Gradually, like some truth drug, the Mandies began to have other side effects. After months of waking at night wracked with fear for no apparent reason, now I began to remember my dreams, dreams that frightened me to the core and left me shaking. I sent Dr Stead long letters describing them in what, for him, must have seemed tediously minute detail. Slowly I was opening up to the past, getting closer to the terror, the nameless darkness inside.

Finally, one dream sent me creeping out of bed to knock urgently on Cathy's door.

"Cathy," I whispered as I opened it a crack. "Are you awake? Can I come in?" Receiving no answer, I opened the door wider and spoke a little louder. "Cathy, can I come in? Do you mind? I've had the most horrible dream!" My voice quavered. "I've got to share it with someone."

Cathy, heavily sedated, replied with an unenthusiastic grunt.

I switched on the light. "I don't know what it means," I said, frightened as a child, as I dragged a chair over to her bedside. "I wanted to shout for help—but I couldn't. Nothing came out. I still remember it so vividly. Maybe it's the Mandies?"

I looked down at Cathy, eyes pleading.

Relenting, she rolled over on her side and, reaching out, took my hand. "So tell us. What 'appened?"

My voice cracked as I repeated myself, forcing back my tears. "I was terrified! There was this big, tough-looking man, maybe in his forties, dressed all in black like an undertaker. But he wasn't an undertaker, Cathy, I knew he wasn't. He was a murderer. He was there to kill me. I knew it as I know you're lying there." And I looked hard at Cathy for emphasis.

"He was standing on this wide runway underneath the wing of a private jet. I was walking past when suddenly he grabbed me and, as he did so, the jets began to whirl—soundlessly. The whole dream was silent. And then this man swung me in the air above him and, with superhuman strength, carried me, headfirst, towards one of the engines. He was going to feed me into the cowling! Chop me up into little bits. I had to scream! To stop him. To hit him. To get help. But I couldn't move. I literally couldn't move. No sound came out. There was nothing but silence!"

I clutched Cathy's hand tightly. "Then I woke up. Sweating. Shaking all over. He was going to kill me, Cathy, I know he was! Or maybe rape me? I don't know. I couldn't scream! It was horrendous. I couldn't scream! Couldn't move. Couldn't defend myself. I was paralysed. It was horrible, horrible, horrible." And I broke down, sobbing great shuddering sobs, struggling to catch my breath.

Cathy withdrew her hand and shifted once more onto her back, gazing up at the ceiling. "Dad often raped me as a kid," she said in her deadened, disconnected voice. "Even before puberty. He'd come into our girls' room. Always drunk. Raped us. I was young. Half thought it was normal—but knew it wasn't really. Never dared tell. Too ashamed." And she rolled back to face me again.

Leaning closer, I took both her hands between mine. "Oh lovey, that's awful! Your dad drunk and inside you? That's just disgusting. It must have been terrifying. And yes, shaming! I can understand that."

Ashamed. Too ashamed. With my inhibitions sliding away, maybe freed by the Mandies, that beast, deep down in the darkest depth of my being, stirred. Raised its head. I suddenly knew for certain, it had to do with rape. And shame.

"You know," I said in a voice full of wonder, "I think you've helped me Cathy, helped me remember something! Something very important is coming back. Rape! You said you never dared tell anyone. You were too ashamed?"

"That's right. It was just me and me sister as knew. Maybe the others, too, but no one said. No one tried to help. Not even our mum. We were all too afraid, see. All afraid of him. Over the years, I just put it to the back of me mind. Till you mentioned it now."

"Did you feel bad about it? Did it make you feel evil?"

"Evil? No. Dirty, diseased, yes."

"I feel evil. All the time. Deeply evil. Like I've got to kill myself. *Got* to. Wipe myself out. Yet I've never known why. But I think this might be it! I think that's maybe where the evil comes from. Nothing to do with dying patients. What if I feel driven to kill myself because instead of dying, I let myself be raped? That horrible dream, just now, it was somehow to do with rape too."

Memories I'd so long managed to keep buried were flooding back, vile memories. And flooding back because I knew I could trust Cathy. That she'd never tell. That I could share anything with her. Nothing I could say would ever shock her. Not Cathy. Not poor Cathy who had seen it all.

Bent over, I clutched my head trying to squeeze those memories to oblivion. Finally, I broke down again in tears, shaking. "Hold me tight Cathy! Please hold me!"

Cathy sat up, reached out to me and wrapped a strong, consoling arm around my heaving shoulders. "It's okay, Clare. It's okay. Really," she murmured. "Tell me. You know I won't say a word. Not to anyone."

I paused as I tried to sort out the splintered shards of memory now ripping through my consciousness, to force them into some sort of coherence. Oh God! Why oh why did I get into his van? All that stupid altruistic stuff I was so full of then.

Dragging the memory out of the dark, black, stinking sludge, I began to put it into words, give it shape, explain as much as I could to Cathy—and to myself.

"I think it was partly the way he asked me. To go for a drink with him, I mean. It wasn't a casual, chat-up line, 'Care for a drink,' sort of thing. At first I said 'No' but then he seemed somehow desperate, vulnerable. He pleaded for me to go with him. And I gave in. After all, Cathy, one glass of wine to keep him company and then home couldn't do any harm, could it? And might somehow help him. " I shifted to look my dear friend in the eyes. She nodded in understanding.

"You know, his van was pretty beat-up. Sort of biscuit coloured. Odd. Different. He had to jerk the door open for me to climb in. It screeched like tortured metal. I can hear it now. And he'd got these big hands." I paused. "He said we'd go to a new place he'd found. It even sounded quite fun. We'd go for a drink. We'd talk and then he'd drive me home."

I felt my eyes tear up with despair. "But it wasn't like that at all. Oh my God! Not at all. First the fog came down. I've had a terror of fog ever since, as a child, I watched that murder film, *Footsteps in the Fog* with a man bludgeoning a woman to death from behind. I had nightmares about it for ages afterwards. And now it was me who was in the fog. Do you see? With a stranger. Where was he taking me? To bludgeon me to death too? The streetlights disappeared. He couldn't be going to a pub! I begged him to take me home; I had to be back by midnight. He replied, I remember it now as if it was yesterday, 'Don't worry, Cinderella, this 'ere's a short cut. You'll get back okay.' Then the van bounded up the kerb. I flew forward, grabbed the dashboard. We jolted across rough ground and came to a halt beside some trees and bushes. 'Where are we?' I heard my voice high, almost shrieking, gripped tight with fear as my eyes darted around the blackness. 'Where've you taken me?' 'Hampstead Heath mi' lovely!' he said. And switched off the engine.

Hampstead Heath, Cathy! The place where murderers dump dead bodies. The man had abducted me and now he was going to murder me."

I began to whimper again. "Murder me in the fog where no one could see. I grabbed hold of the door handle and jerked it hard. It wouldn't budge! I pounded and pounded it. Ah!"

I paused. Turned to Cathy, eyes wide with sudden insight. "Maybe that's why I'm so afraid of closed doors! They threaten to trap me. I felt him lean towards me in the dark, Cathy, his breath in my ear. Then he put his hands around my neck. Look, like this!" I lifted my hands to my neck to demonstrate. "And then he gently squeezed. 'Now get in the back!' he hissed. I still remember his hands. They were long-fingered, quite warm, though it was cold outside. I should have shouted. Oh Cathy, of course I should have shouted but I was afraid he'd kill me, throttle me, just to shut me up. And who would have heard me anyway? No one. There was no one there but him and me and the fog. I did as he told me. I climbed through into the back. And there was a blanket rolled up on the floor. Why had he got a blanket on the floor? Did he do this often? Was it waiting for me? Was he a serial rapist or murderer, or both? Had he planned this all along and here was me, the naïve little virgin, who fell into his trap?" I drew in a shuddering breath.

"It's not your fault, Clare. It's not." Cathy took a tissue from her locker and wiped away my tears and then handed me the hanky to blow my nose. "Did you tell the police?"

My sobs abated. "No! I didn't tell anyone," I sniffed. "Not a soul. Not till now. You're the first person I've ever told. I'd buried it don't you see. Until that dream and you talking of rape, I'd never remembered anything at all until now. I suppose I was just so ashamed of my own stupidity. Me, who liked to consider myself bright. I couldn't face it. I must have buried it deep, deep down inside me and covered it with a heavy slab of shame and guilt." I twisted out of Cathy's hold and slumped back in the chair, eyes down, looking at my fingers.

My voice came out muffled now, almost as if I couldn't let the words squeeze past my lips. "I lay there on his blanket. Stiff as a board. Thighs clenched tight together. But Hey!" I raised my head to look at Cathy. "I've just realised, that was when I had my first out-of-body experience. You remember I told you about them. It must have been terror that drove me to a place hard up against the van's ceiling, staring down on what looked like my dead body. Perhaps even my ghost? I watched remotely as, one by one, he undid the buttons of my blouse, pulled up my bra, fondled my breasts.

Then he ordered me to touch him—and I came back to earth. I thought he meant touch his chest. How laughable and innocent is that? It was all thick matted hair. But of course that's not what he meant at all. He grabbed my hand and forced it further down. His fly was already open. He'd got no underwear on, and his penis was hard and huge. He rolled on top of me. He was so heavy, Cathy, he forced the breath out of me. I could feel the corrugated metal of the van's floor pressing into my spine. He groaned and thrust and shuddered—and then he came." I shivered then felt the blood drain from my face, go pale with shame. "He came, withdrew and jerked off in my belly button, his sticky semen overflowing down my side! Maybe that's why I can't bear anyone to touch me there, even doctors."

After a long silence I lifted my head and looked at my friend. "And yet men seem to think being raped is nothing. Just sex without the love. I've been in hell for two years, Cathy, my whole character's changed. I used to be so full of joy! Instead I've felt filthy, diseased, evil. I've tried to kill myself three times, do you realise that? Tried to rid the world of my 'wickedness'. Being raped and that terror of being murdered, that will probably scar me for the rest of my life. If, that is, I go on living."

"How did you get away?"

"How did I get away?" I paused to think. How *did* I get away?

"That's really bizarre. I don't know. I don't know. Was I so zombied that I registered nothing?"

As I thought more I said, "I think I remember reaching a white, panelled, front door. Was that the nurses' hostel? It was night. But how did I get there? Had I walked in the dark? Hitch-hiked? Did he drive me?

Surely not! Indeed, how did I get out of the van? Did he open the door? Dump me at the roadside? Was there a late-night bus?"

I sat silent for a while, trying to take in what I had revealed. Trying to attach it to my self. Then I stood up.

"What are you going to do now?" Cathy asked.

"Go back to bed I suppose. I'm shattered. I'm sorry I woke you, Cath, but thanks so much for listening. You're such a good friend!" And I stroked Cathy's hand with my fingertips and walked towards the door.

When I woke the next morning, I lay quite still, staring at the ceiling, slowly picking over what had happened in the night. I searched my psyche to see whether somehow those revelations had changed how I felt about myself, my essence. But I found no change. Indeed, the black beast that I had watched creeping towards me over the past weeks was almost upon me. And then there was the shame. Partly shame at not having dared to scream, not having fought more but also at being so utterly stupid as to get into the man's van in the first place.

The morning after the revelation, I dressed myself in my black polo-necked sweater and black miniskirt, those birthday presents from my beloved mother. This way I'd have her wrapped close around me to the end.

I waited until the afternoon medicines had been handed out and then I headed up to my room. I brought out the beautiful black and gold powder compact from its hiding place, prised off the tray of powder and took out the hidden blade. I had decided to do a venous cut-down, a procedure doctors sometimes performed in an emergency to access large veins in patients in shock when their peripheral veins had collapsed. I'd tried cutting my wrists months ago, but I didn't bleed enough. This time I would go for a big vein. And this time it had to work.

I lay down on top of the bed and started to cut. It hurt far more than I'd expected as I sliced down through the flesh searching, searching for that vein. I paused and peered and then took a deep breath, gritted my teeth and cut down some more until at last there it was, dark venous blood welling up over my razor blade, warm and sticky over my fingers. In relief I lay back and relaxed watching my life blood oozing from me.

But venous blood, though conveniently available, flows more slowly and clots more quickly than its arterial sister, so time and again I had to use the razor to keep the red stream draining from me.

After a while I began to feel thirsty. Then the thirst grew—and grew. Eventually it obsessed me more than the pain or the blood which now covered both my hands and had somehow wiped off on my face and dried, shrivelling up my skin as it did so. My clothes lay heavy with the blood's weight, the dent in the mattress beside my hip, a dark pool. But it was the thirst that cried out. The room had no basin. I would have to go to the bathroom. I *had* to drink. Cautiously I sat up and lowered myself out of bed. My head swam but I held on, regained my balance and set out with my empty glass for the door. Looking back, I saw a growing puddle of blood under the bed, blood working its way, drip by drip through the mattress. It was going to work! Surely this time it would work. Soon the world would be rid of me forever. And I of it.

As I opened the door I glanced cautiously left and right, ready to pull back at the first sign of anyone in the corridor. But there was no one and the bathrooms lay just across the way. Tiptoeing, I made it to a tap, filled the glass, drank it and then drank another and another and then filled the glass again and headed back to my bed. Vaguely my enfeebled brain noticed splashes of blood on the corridor floor but by now I was losing consciousness, my head fuzzy and my ears full of noise. I had to get back to bed and quickly.

From a semi-conscious world, I felt someone shaking me, trying to rouse me. She searched for my pulse. Briefly I came to as they lifted me onto a stretcher. Sister Garrett had hold of my hand.

"Oh Clare darlin' why didn't you tell us? You could surely have told us that you needed help?"

In all they gave me six pints of blood and plasma at the hospital and put eight stitches in the cut. Slowly my brain recovered from its oxygen starvation and consciousness returned.

The first person to appear beside my bed was my mother. *Oh no, poor Mum. What have you ever done to deserve all this? Nothing! I was trying to save you don't you see? To save you and the world.* A single tear seeped from the corner of my eye. I felt it creep slowly down my cheek and then my neck but didn't have the energy to wipe it away.

Later Dr Stead looked down sadly at my drained face on the pillow. This was the end of the road for us. I knew it was coming. It wasn't fair to the staff or patients to keep me in the Villa. On my discharge I'd be heading to St Francis where he would lose touch with me for, although he was director of all the county's psychiatric services, he kept no beds for his patients in St Francis's long-term asylum. After all, few there received psychiatric treatment or were expected to get better. Basically, I had failed us both.

18

The Main Building Where Serendipity Unfolds

ARRIVING BACK AT the Villa from hospital, I discovered that Cathy had been transferred to the Main Building. Now I was to join her. After packing my few things into holdalls, Sister Garrett turned to a couple of white-coated male nurses, handed the bags to one and my hospital records to the other.

"They're waiting for Clare in the Women's Closed Ward. You can take the path through the coppice if you like," and she gave me a final smile. We wouldn't be seeing each other again.

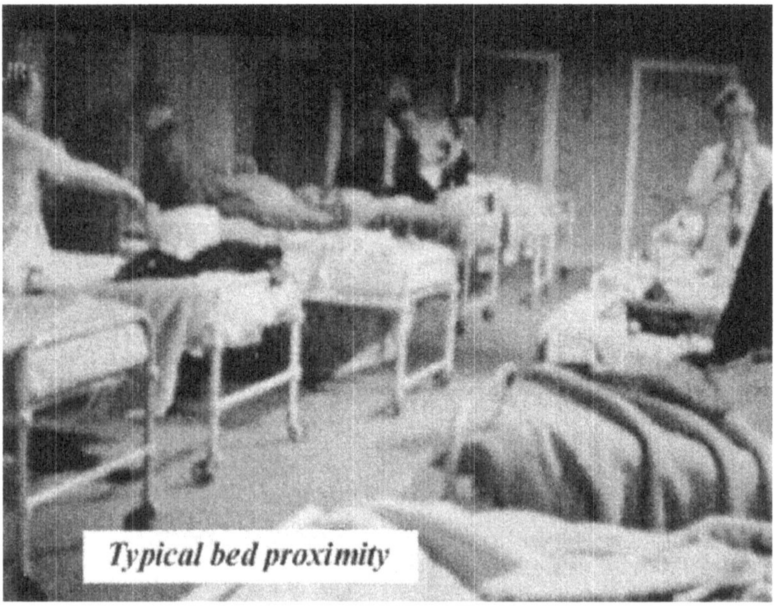

Overcrowding at St Francis, late 1960s. [Credit: Joe Hughes]

Research shows that, in 1859, St Francis had officially opened under its first superintendent, Dr Charles Lockhart Robinson. A world pioneer in the field of mental health, he was totally against the then common practice of treating the mentally sick as little better than animals. Instead of keeping them shackled, he offered patients respect. The great meadows of my time were part of the ethos of St Francis, as Dr Robinson incorporated farming experience on the 119-acre estate into the rehabilitation of male patients. He even organised calming Turkish baths for his female patients—and with successful results. A man a century ahead of his time, Dr Robinson and his innovative adoption of the non-restraint of patients attracted medical visitors from all over Europe. Sadly, by the time I reached the place, Robinson's pioneering spirit had been stifled long ago by lack of funds.[xxxv]

A heavy key ground in the lock on the far side of the door. Sister Powell, large bosom and greying moustache to the fore, ushered us in.

The first thing to hit me was the smell. The stink of urine permeated the air. Pausing a moment, I gazed desolately down the long length of beds. Then a nurse moved me on past an elderly patient huddling behind a chair, moaning softly as she swayed herself back and forth in thrall to some inner pain.

I'd arrived at rock bottom. This was where the incurably insane were stockpiled, the old, the demented. Only Cathy and I were young. None of us was expected to go anywhere soon—if ever. Sister led me to one of a row of overflow beds placed in a corridor facing the washrooms and told me to change into a hospital gown.

That night I wrote one last note to Dr Stead.

Oh bury me not on the lone prairie
Where coyotes howl and the wind blows free.
Oh bury me not, but my voice failed there
For you took no heed of my dying prayer.
In a narrow bed just six by three
You buried me there on the lone prairie

The senior registrar, Dr Kozlov,[xxxvi] was sitting in a little cubbyhole off the main ward and, throughout my brief interview, she kept the door open. Was it for ventilation or was she afraid of being attacked? Patient antipathy towards her was almost tangible. Not contempt, like patients had at The Lady Chich for Dr Hallow. Dr Kozlov was not stupid or obsessed. She was, quite simply, malicious. I scanned her eyes, the lines around her mouth, searching for some kindlier characteristic but found none.

My problem was that I had to break through that stony barrier. I had to have a prescription for DF118. I asked for them as pleasantly as I could, but I needn't have bothered. Dr Kozlov turned the request down flat. "I never prescribe any medicine except Largactil during the day and a mild sedative at night. I see no reason why I should change a life-long policy just for you, Miss Thompson. Do you?"

Next day I was sent for by the administrative director of the hospital, Dr Wheeler.[xxxvii] Strictly speaking, I was his patient, but I would be sharing him with some one hundred and fifty others.

"Good morning, Clare. Please sit down. I'll go straight to the point. St Francis is quite different to the clinics you've been used to in the past. We don't believe in deep psychotherapy here and depend instead on rest and occupational therapy to help people feel better." I'm sure he sincerely believed that theirs was the best cure for most mental illness. In some cases, such as Cathy's and maybe even mine, I think he was right. "Is there any more I can do for you?"

I seized my chance. "Yes, there is one thing. I have this pain in my arm. At the Villa I took DF118 three times a day. For the first time in years I was able to sleep without pain while normal chloral hydrate doesn't touch me at all. And I *must* sleep." Alarm was creeping into my voice. "And one other thing: ward conferences terrify me."

"Right. Well, I'll see what I can do with the conference and I'll have a word with Sister about the pills." Standing, he gathered up his papers. "I hope you'll settle in soon, Clare. Once you get used to our methods I think you'll find that they'll help you a lot." And he ushered me out of his office.

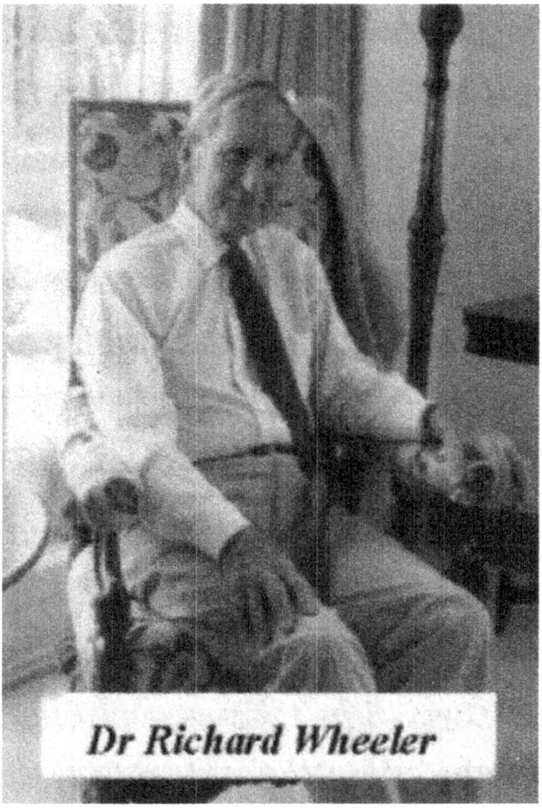

Dr Richard Wheeler, physician superintendent,
St Francis Hospital. [Credit: Joe Hughes]

Two days later Dr Wheeler held his weekly ward conference. Patients were moved off the radiators and the floor where they liked to sit leaning against the walls, periodically softly peeing into their adult nappies.

Would he send for me after all? Had the moment I'd been dreading arrived?

A nurse called me in. Pot plants had been dragged into the sitting area to lend a touch of gentility, but the basic concept was the same. One patient pitted against an assortment of staff. Tight-lipped and seething inside, I endured in silence but, once dismissed, my anger exploded.

Looking round I spied a locker. With one sweep of my arm I sent flying the jug and glass that graced its top, shouting, "He promised, the bastard, he promised!"

Boy! It felt good. Harsh, bitter words spat between clenched teeth. Power flowed into my body and I turned to look for some other inanimate victim for my fury. Gone was the desolation of betrayal, replaced by hate, good honest hate. A hate and anger that I had so long denied because Christ had said, "Thou shalt love thy neighbour as thy self."

"Okay God!" I shouted. "I hate myself don't I? So why shouldn't I hate them too? What are you going to do about it? Huh? Send me to Hell? I'm already there!" I hurled the words out as if to reach the roof of the world and pound at the Almighty's barred gates.

But then a strange thing happened. Before the nurses, scurrying in from the conference, had time to reach me, Cathy appeared. For a moment I fought her too, but Cathy held me tight. "Clare, stop!" she whispered, "Don't let 'em get you. They'll send you to Disturbed.[xxxviii] They can do anythin'. Just hush. Hush, baby." And Cathy held me so I couldn't escape, and rocked me so I would feel safe, as she had no doubt rocked her little children months before.

As she did so, all the fight drained from me as the waves on the seashore drain down into the sand. Slowly great sobs began to wrack my body as I leant against my friend, buried my face in her shoulder and realised once and for all that I was locked in and could not escape.

Released from Cathy's embrace, I turned in vain to the windows behind my bed. Windows which mocked me, letting me see out, tempting me to freedom whilst locking me in. These were high, Victorian windows that didn't open, divided into many small panes by wooden glazing bars.

I lifted a hand and in a final act of despair, punched at one of the panes. To my amazement it broke! (In the Villa the windows had been reinforced against suicide; I knew, I'd tried them.) But now those old-fashioned, ten-inch squares of glass popped like paper bags under my fists. As the glass broke so too did something inside me; all the frustrations and anger as well as the fear and loneliness of fighting single-handedly against the monolithic, 1960's psychiatric system, was suddenly set free. I had broken at least a dozen before they wrenched me clear and lifted me, still struggling, onto the bed.

As one nurse laid himself heavily across my body, pinning me down, another bared my arm and thrust the sedative deep into my vein.

Slowly I got to know my fellow inmates. A cheery old lady in her late eighties, universally known as the 'Duchess', had become a sort of ward mascot. She shuffled up and down through the rooms in decrepit slippers and a shabby dressing gown, a shoe box tucked under her arm. She came over to my bed in the corridor and, pointing at the box, asked in a kindly voice, "Have you met my dog, Sammy?" At mealtimes she fed 'Sammy' with scraps from her plate. At night, the staff cleaned out the box, lined it with fresh newspaper and returned it to the place under the Duchesses bed where, she claimed, Sammy slept best. The Duchess lived a life full of joyful surprises. When the inmates watched the Grand National on the ward television, it was her husband, 'the Duke', whose horse won. The old lady rejoiced enthusiastically and a good portion of the patients with her. One fateful day she reported that her husband's chauffeur had accidentally run the Rolls into the ship, the *Queen Mary*—but there now, as he owned both, it was no great cause for concern. Of the forty-odd patients I quickly decided that, apart from Cathy, I liked the 'Duchess of Normandy' best.

A few days after my arrival, a frisson of excitement ran through the staff, and was quickly picked up by their more lucid patients. The nurses had received special instructions about a new admission. The patient, said to be in her thirties, had been consigned by a local judge to the Women's Closed Ward for mental assessment and observation. According to rumour, she and her boyfriend, both drug addicts and desperate for a fix, had gone out one evening to a corner shop. The woman had hit the elderly owner over the head with a wooden cosh while her partner stole a pathetic few pounds from the till. The two had fled, leaving their victim bleeding on the floor, later to die of her injuries. Observing the murderess from afar, it struck me how essentially normal she looked.

In contrast to Mrs Roberts. A severe, closed-faced woman, she was never called by her first name and had been confined in the locked ward for almost two years. Her problems had all begun when her husband died suddenly of a heart attack. The poor woman had become acutely distressed and had started accosting everyone she met—in shops, cinemas and at tea parties—telling them that she was a whore, an evil prostitute, street filth, and should be jailed. Her adult children urgently sought help from a psychiatrist and he in turn sent her, sectioned, to our ward for treatment. A course of ECT did nothing to help her, while even heavy doses of Largatil failed to ease her anguish. Finally, after considerable consultation between family and medical staff, they decided to subject her to a lobotomy, severing most of the connections between her frontal lobes and the rest of her brain.

The purpose was to reduce her symptoms of severe mental distress. And, on that basis, one could say that it worked. However, the brain's frontal lobes are vitally involved in human personality. They influence spontaneity, judgement, problem solving, memory, language, impulse control, and social and sexual behaviour. Sever them and the patient's whole character is changed.

At the height of its popularity, in one year alone, some 20,000 patients in the United States were lobotomised and, in Ontario, Canada, around 74% of lobotomies were performed on women, a gender bias similar to the number of cases of hypochondriasis diagnosed by male doctors about female patients, as I knew to my cost. It was doctors in the Soviet Union who concluded that the procedure was "contrary to the principles of humanity" and that "through lobotomy an insane person is changed into an idiot."

Instantly after her operation, Mrs Roberts's outward torment vanished. Instead her children were left with a stranger; a woman emotionally blunted, suffering from inertia, totally lacking in empathy or the ability to care and love. At the same time, she had also lost all inhibitions and we fellow patients listened gleefully as she told Dr Kozlov, in no uncertain terms, exactly what she thought of her; things that the rest of us only dared mutter behind the woman's back for fear of retaliation.

One ray of brightness in that dreary ward was that Dr Wheeler was taking an interest in Cathy's case. On the very first day we were reunited, Cathy turned to me, smiling broadly, and said, "Shall I make you coffee? I can, you know. The voices are much quieter."

Apparently, in reviewing her family background, Dr Wheeler had made a link between her husband's violent abandonment, the birth of her fifth child and the onset of hallucinations, later made worse by the removal of all five of her young children. He had told Cathy that he believed she could be helped by complete rest and freedom from stress. That her diagnosis of schizophrenia might be incorrect. He gave orders for her to be allowed to stay on the ward instead of going to occupational therapy and said that any of Cathy's requests, within reason, were to be granted. It now appeared that Dr Wheeler's plans were bearing fruit.

But then Dr Wheeler announced he was taking a month's sabbatical. Cathy came in search of me. "He called me into his office. Asked me how I was doin'. How were the voices. I told him that they were better, less demandin'. And then I told him how I'd managed to make you a cup of coffee!" and Cathy smiled at me with gentle satisfaction. "He sounded real pleased. Then he told me that, while he was away, he wanted me to continue as I have been and that the most important thing for me was rest. Relax he said. Try not to worry about anythin'. You know, Clare, he really seemed as if he cared. A man who really cared!" Cathy sounded slightly dazed at the idea. "At the end he said he'd be back very soon and that, if I need anythin' I can ask Dr Kozlov. He must be joking! I'd never ask that woman for anythin' in a hundred years."

A week later Dr Kozlov sent for Cathy. Told her that she was being moved out of the locked ward and up to the gallery. I visited the gallery once when Cathy was there. Left over from the 19th century, it consisted of a corridor of tiny, cell-like rooms in the attic. Their furnishings comprised one low cot bed, one small cupboard and a hard, upright chair. Nothing more. Oh, and each room still retained its original spyhole in the door.

Cathy returned, deeply distressed. "Dr Kozlov said the opposite of everythin' Dr Wheeler had told me. Said as I must go to occupational therapy. That I can't sit around in the ward for the rest of me life. And at the end she said she's goin' to discharge me very soon. Clare, I can't do it! I can't survive out there! Not yet. I told 'er Dr Wheeler said as I wasn't to have any worries, any stress. She just said flat that Dr Wheeler had left me in her care and it was up to her to decide. Clare, out there it'll kill me, truly it will!"

I tried speaking to Sister Powell, but she said there was nothing she could do to stop Cathy's release and, sure enough, before Dr Wheeler returned, Cathy had been discharged. It all happened so quickly she didn't even have time to get permission to enter the locked ward and say goodbye to me.

I, meanwhile, was slowly slipping into a drugged stupor. No longer violent, I was moved into a four-bedded side ward. Unable to think—unable to cause trouble—I lay mute, inert, out of contact with the world for months, I don't know exactly how long; a silent shadow. I'd given up. I no longer tried to fight the system. No longer interacted with the staff or patients. I lay on my bed waiting for the Apocalypse. Did anyone notice? I don't remember. After all, their job was to keep the patients safe, clean and fed. No one in the Main Building was expected to be cured. Finally, my oft repeated request had been answered: they left me alone. I remembered then Dr Wheeler's words when I arrived. That, instead of psychotherapy, St Francis depended on rest and occupational therapy to help people feel better. Maybe, as with Cathy, it would work.

Then something strange happened. Slowly, mysteriously pale shoots of new life stirred somewhere inside my mind. I heard a 'voice', surely in truth my own thoughts, saying, *What in the world do you think you're doing lying there? Do you imagine angels are going to swoop down, wrap you in their wings and carry you over the high walls to freedom? If you want to get out of here you better do something about it yourself.*

And I sat up and looked around.

For the first time in months, I took in my surroundings. Saw the plain annex and its four beds, each in its own corner of the room, coupled to a bedside locker and armchair. Auspiciously, the sun came shining in through the window. The room was empty, the other three inmates away at occupational therapy. Probably weaving ruddy baskets, I thought cynically. Yes, cynicism, too, had returned.

Then something caught my eye. A newspaper lay abandoned on the floor by a neighbour's bed. I gazed at it—and reckoned it must be half a year since I last read anything.

Urged on by this strange new appetite for life, I climbed off my bed, picked up the newspaper and sat down in the nearest chair. My concentration already shot and starting at the back, I flicked absently through the *Sunday Express*'s pages. Then, abruptly, a headline broke through the fog of medication. *"Home is a lone boat to Edward Allcard."* Lone? What heavenly fantasy was this? Sharing life with a ward full of sectioned psychiatric patients was never exactly quiet, peaceful, 'alone'. There's a big difference between being alone and being lonely. I often felt lonely, as if there was no one on my side, no one seeing life—death—my way. Whereas being alone was a silent luxury which lunatic asylums seldom granted you—unless you were in a padded cell.

I read on.

According to the article, Edward Allcard was halfway through a solo circumnavigation of the world—something very unusual in those days (though Francis Chichester was to follow him around Cape Horn some months later). In 1957, Allcard and his friend Peter Tangvald had been the first ever to race single-handed east to west across the Atlantic—the prize, one dollar, won by Peter. Now, ten years later, Allcard had left his yacht, *Sea Wanderer*, moored in Auckland harbour, New Zealand, and had flown back to be with his recently widowed mother, who was herself dying.

The interviewing journalist reported, "He is friendly and surprisingly easy to talk to yet there is undoubtedly something of the recluse about him..." Questioned about this, Allcard replied:

"Yes, I do consider myself anti-social but, wherever I go in the world, I have friends—an enormous number of friends. Of course, the ideal would be to have a girl with the same idea to come along too..."

Finishing the article, I lowered the paper and sat for a long time thinking. *Freedom! Adventure! That's what the man's got. Personal freedom to roam the world at will. To follow his dreams. Never having to ask permission from anyone. No metal locks and high stone walls shutting him in.* My drugged heartbeat quickened at the mere thought of it.

Getting slowly to my feet, I wandered out of the side ward to the nurses' station in search of pencil, paper and envelope. I would write the man a letter. Maybe he would rescue me?

Dear Mr Allcard,

I've just read the *Sunday Express*'s interview about you sailing alone around the world. How wonderful! In it you said the ideal would be to find a girl with the same idea to go along too.

Well, I'm 22. I'm afraid I can't actually sail or cook and am nothing much to look at, but I can swim and speak French and, to me, your way of life sounds absolutely perfect. I'd love to go with you. There's just one small problem. Right now I'm locked up in a loony bin and they probably won't let me out till November. Could you wait that long before leaving?

I look forward to hearing from you.

Yours sincerely

Clare Thompson

Sealing the envelope, I addressed it to Edward Allcard Esq, c/o The *Sunday Express*, Fleet Street, London and, begging a stamp from the nurses' station, asked them to post it.

Then I climbed back onto my bed to think. It was as if those past months without treatment, without delving into my failings as a human being either by them or myself, had somehow nurtured seeds of healing. Could it be that I was not so powerfully evil after all? It was as if the article had somehow awakened me from a deep sleep. Maybe out there, I still had a chance of life, even adventure?

I dreamed on. *What do I do next? If he replies? I can't even remember where to begin. I suppose I have to persuade Wheeler to set me free. Can he cancel my Section? How does it work? How long was the Section for in the first place? A year until November? Or was it open-ended? Who can I ask?*

With my newfound hunger for life, I noticed that, as dark depression slowly receded, the Largactil haze proved easier to overcome.

As soon as Dr Wheeler returned, I initiated the next step in my strategy. I wrote another letter, this time to him. In it, all my pent-up anger against confinement, against forced treatments, the institution of psychiatry itself and its sexist singling out of women, flooded out.

Dear Dr Wheeler,

Please can I see you. I want your permission to leave. I see it like this.

During the sixteenth century, the Inquisition—priests—men—hunted down women who did not conform to society's norms. The priests labelled the women witches. Scapegoats for society's ills, these women were imprisoned and interrogated. They were alternately sweet-talked and tortured for as long as it took them to confess to their crime of witchcraft. The Inquisition then burnt them anyway, their own consciences now clear.

Today, in the 1960s, psychiatrists, usually men, treat patients, more often women, who in some way do not conform to accepted norms. For instance, I happen to believe that, when life is dominated by pain, it is better to be dead. Others believe they hear voices.

Encouraged by an embarrassed society, psychiatrists lock us away, alternately sweet-talking and torturing us, or at least subjecting us to ECT and deep narcosis, until, sooner or later, we confess to our crime of mental illness. (Was it perhaps the psychiatrists that drove us mad in the first place?) Claiming to help us, they are in fact following a darker agenda: to destroy our unacceptable differences.

I've been held in psychiatric units for more than two years. I have been given 26 ECTs and 30 days of deep narcosis. I now wish to be set free. I want to go out and find a job and live my own life. Please give me permission to leave.

Yours sincerely

Clare Thompson

Two days later Dr Wheeler sent for me.

"Come in. Sit down." His voice sounded cold as he held up my letter. "I have just received your letter. Let me read it to you." And he proceeded to read it aloud.

Listening to it, I thought two things. First that it was rather well crafted—and second that, read that way, it did sound unnecessarily harsh, not the most sensible way to try to get discharged.

Once finished, Dr Wheeler went on, "I have to say I found this letter both hurtful and ungrateful. We've spent two years and a lot of money trying to keep you alive. Dr Stead, in particular, has shown endless patience, devoting many hours to trying to help you when you were very unhappy and disturbed." He paused and watched me for some reaction.

Whilst I did indeed feel ashamed, I was determined not to recant. Writing that letter in the heat of the moment had proved a cathartic release of two years of frustrations. I conceded that perhaps the months of lying on my bed had provided the stress-free treatment he had recommended; and now I felt I had suddenly woken up from a long nightmare.

"Well, I'm happy to hear that. Truly. This has been a very difficult time not only for you but also for your poor parents. But I must warn you, life's not easy out there. When we admitted you, I expected you to stay here for at least seven years. And really Clare, I don't think you're ready to go out yet. If you go now, I think it very likely that you'll be back again before you're 40—and in a much worse condition. Then you'll be in here for life."

"But I want to try! I can't know till I try. Please let me try. I'm only 22. I could have a whole new life ahead of me. Please!"

Dr Wheeler studied me more closely. It was as if he could see some physical sign of change. Had my deadened eyes come alive? Were they more focussed? Alert? I held his gaze with mine, willing him to agree. It seemed to work.

"Let me make a suggestion. Search the local papers, find one or two jobs you think you could cope with and then I'll give you a day pass to go for interviews. How does that sound?"

I felt my whole face relax. I'd won! I beamed at him in gratitude and stood up. "That would be wonderful! Thank you *so* much. And please, could you cut down on the Largactil? If I'm going to be interviewed, I need to be able to think." I left the room and went in search of a local newspaper.

19

HOPE

IT TOOK ME a little over a week to arrange a couple of job interviews in Brighton, both part-time night nursing in retirement homes. Maybe I'd be able to visit Cathy in her council house at the same time.

A bus ride and short walk delivered me to the first nursing home. I later learnt that the owner was a man who had sold off his string of garages in order to invest in old people. The profits were so much higher.

A middle-aged woman greeted me at the door, her uniform grubby and smelling of cigarettes. I soon discovered that the home served old people with dementia dried egg and instant mashed potato, while those who were *compos mentis*, and able to complain to relatives, received the more expensive and nutritious fresh varieties. To further save money, the nurses themselves were made to deal with the soiled sheets rather than pack them off to a commercial laundry. Each bedroom had a washbasin, which looked good in the brochures sent out to the clients' families—but only cold water ran through the single taps. Despite outer appearances, it was altogether a shocking, cut-rate place.

The second home was the exact opposite. Set in a large Edwardian house with a garden, it represented the retirement dream of Matron Lewis. Every resident was her guest, and her staff were servants dedicated to their comfort. To hammer this idea home, Matron Lewis showed me precisely how one blind resident's breakfast tray should be set up. I remember it to this day. The cup of tea in the upper righthand corner, a glass of fruit juice next to it. Then a carefully cut half of grapefruit in the centre. On the left, fingers of toast and marmalade and on the edge closest to the patient, a linen napkin.

In the summer, the nurses could bring their small children to play in the garden for the old people's enjoyment. After the interview, Matron said to me that if I accepted the job, three nights a week, I had to promise I would stay at least six months, as staff changes unsettled her guests.

With the two interviews for part time work successfully negotiated, I went in search of Cathy. I found the housing estate easily enough. The house was quite large, unsurprisingly so as it was originally intended for her family of seven. I went round the back and knocked on the door. There was no answer. Then I tried the handle. It turned. I pulled up short in the entrance and gazed at the kitchen in disbelief. It was as if the owners were in the last stages of moving house. Almost everything that could have been stripped from the place had been: no fridge, no table and chairs, just a small stove and one saucepan. I called out and heard Cathy answer from upstairs. I found her in bed, huddled under a sheet and one thin blanket. Here, too, everything had vanished: no carpet, no curtains, no bedside table or lamp, no wardrobe or chair. Nothing.

Cathy looked at me, her eyes wide in astonishment and disbelief. As I walked over to her, she gave me a slight, sad smile.

"Cathy, it's me, Clare." And I bent over and gave her a fleeting hug. Then I settled down on the bed beside her, one arm around my dear friend's shoulders, my thoughts flitting back to that time when she had done the same for me.

"Cathy, what's all this about? What's happened? Where has everything gone? Looks like you've been raided by gangsters!"

"I have. Me family. They stole everythin'. First Social stoled me five kids and then me family does this. I've got nothin'." The words came out in Cathy's old, dead voice, her conversation almost monosyllabic. She had lost every tiny shoot of progress Dr Wheeler had tried so hard to nurture. I looked around, seeing the place for the first time through Cathy's eyes, a mother's eyes. Realising that it was here that, for several years, she must have cared for and cuddled and loved her children, raised them as best she could, a house full of voices.

Then I spotted a large plastic container of sleeping pills on the windowsill, picked it up and rattled it. "And where did you get this then?"

"My GP. That's for the next month."

"He must be mad, Cathy! I mean how could he be so stupid?" I carried them over to the bed. "I don't like them sitting here. Love. Not at all. Please let me take some of them with me."

"No, no! Don't do that!" Cathy burst out, snatching them away and burying them under the blanket. "You can't do that! I won't take 'em, Clare, promise. They're just sort of like a guarantee. To make me feel protected. From everything. Family. Everyone."

I took Cathy's cold hands in mine and chafed them, hoping to rub some warmth into them so that it could travel to her heart. "When did you last eat, my love?" I asked gently.

"Don't know." She brought back memories of my empty cupboards in Hove.

"Look. I'll go down and see if I can find something in the kitchen. If not, is there a shop nearby?"

"Yeah. Back door. Round the corner. To the left."

"Right, you stay here, and I'll see what I can find. We can have lunch together, but then I've got to go back."

The first thing I did on my return to St Francis was search out Nurse George, in my opinion the most efficient of the ward's elderly nurses. In one of the little consulting rooms, I told her what I'd found, making sure she was grasping the full significance of it. "I wanted to take the pills away. She said her GP prescribed them, but I simply can't believe it. A month of sleeping pills for a woman just out of psychiatric hospital? She promised she wouldn't take an overdose, but I don't trust her."

"Understood. I'll get onto it right away."

"Please! I feel really awful. I know I should have taken them away whatever she said. But after everything else had been stripped from her, it seemed too cruel. I thought she might hang herself. But, Nurse, someone must go and see her right now. *Today.* Tomorrow could be too late. Or why not ring straight away for an ambulance to take her to hospital?"

It was three days later that I heard Cathy had been found dead the next morning by a health visitor sent round to check on her. I was torn apart: fury, guilt, desolation. Why hadn't they done as I said? Was it because I was a patient? Why didn't they go to her at once? Wasn't Cathy's life worth the bother? And why for God sakes hadn't I just fought her for the pills? Cathy, who had been so good to me, so kind. Still, for once, I didn't entirely blame myself. In my opinion it was Dr Kozlov who had Cathy's death on her hands.

The following day, I went again to see Dr Wheeler. I told him about my meeting with Cathy, how I'd begged for someone to see her and then presented him with my two letters for part-time employment: two nights a week with the Garage Man on top of the three nights a week offered by Matron Lewis. Somewhat reluctantly, Dr Wheeler cancelled my Section.

I was going to be allowed another chance at making it outside. And this time it felt different. This time I wasn't forcing myself as a duty, or as a way of manoeuvring towards killing myself. No black clouds lurked on the horizon. This time I *wanted* to succeed. This time life was luring me out with extraordinary fantasies.

*   *   *

Two hours' drive away in a country cottage in Hampshire, the single-handed sailor Edward Allcard used a paperknife to slit open the small brown envelope. He told me later that he had felt mildly alarmed to get yet another letter forwarded by the *Sunday Express*. For mine was not the first he had received in response to his offhand remark in that interview, where he'd said the ideal would be to find a girl with the same idea. In the past he'd quite often regretted words he'd said in an unguarded moment to the press, which was one of the reasons he did his best to avoid them. After all, his present ambition was to sail single-handed around the world and such plans held no room for a second person.

Pulling out the note, he remarked that it had been written in pencil on lined white paper. But it was the words themselves, their honesty, that caught his attention and touched his heart. He prized personal freedom above everything and here was a young woman locked up by the state in a lunatic asylum.

He sat for a long time at his sister's cottage window, gazing out over the fields below, while he decided how to reply.

A few days later I received this.

21st April, 1968

Dear Clare (if I may call you that)

Thank you very much for your message which eventually reached me via the *Sunday Express*. I both appreciate your offer and the honesty of your letter.

Oddly enough a close friend of mine suffered a similar nervous breakdown and had to undergo psychiatric treatment. She came out of hospital quite cured, which is usual these days. The doctors get plenty of practice! And you have the advantage of youth, 22 you say. I am over double your age, but I feel I understand you. You sound a very interesting girl, so hurry up and get well again. I think you would find an ocean voyage monotonous, but when I am nearer an interesting cruising ground, I would consider it an honour to take you for a trip.

Best wishes,

Edward Allcard

Honour! He would consider it an Honour to have me to come along too? Me, a freak, a nutcase, did he know, even for a moment, what that incredibly kind word meant to me?

Having found work and been discharged from hospital, once again my faithful parents came to the rescue. They discovered a tiny attic bedsit in Hove, Sussex, with a shared bathroom on the next landing down. I loved it. The ceiling sloped so low that I had to be careful not to bang my head as I sat up in the morning. I had a little dormer window that looked out over the rooftops to the sea. It reminded me of one of my favourite children's books, *A Little Princess*.

As with most new jobs, the first week was the worst. After being silent for so long, I had to relearn how to chat to people, to look them in the eye, to smile reassuringly. Luckily, I was on nights when the patients were mostly asleep. Bit by bit I pieced together why each elderly patient had ended up in a home. Some had fallen, broken a hip and found it impossible to regain their independence. Some were going blind. Some had dementia, their elderly spouses unable to cope with them any longer. Those of our clients with purely physical problems often found the lack of mental stimulation in the homes, the loss of freedom and variety in their lives, very hard to bear and would slide into depression. Visits from friends and family were their lifelines.

Meanwhile, I began tentatively to put out feelers towards the world. Working nights meant I had all day to sleep and explore. I bought a sun lounger and carried it down my narrow street to the beach, there to snooze away sunny mornings. I tried cinemas and waterfront cafés. Nursing, too, was bringing satisfaction. I hadn't been working in the Garage Man's Home more than a few days when I was asked to blanket bath a new patient. Her nearest relatives, a nephew and niece, had just moved her to us from a previous care home.

As I approached her bed with a trolley laden with soap, a basin of hot water and towel, the old lady began to whimper, "Please don't touch my leg. Please not!"

With the top sheet stripped back, I looked at her thin, dry-skinned legs—and noticed at once that one leg was shorter than the other.

"Has your right leg always been shorter?"

"Is it shorter? I don't know. I don't remember. They dropped me out of bed at the other place, and it still hurts."

I went at once in search of Sister. Previously noted for my sharp powers of observation, it was good to find I hadn't lost my talent. Sister called an ambulance right away. The old woman was operated on the following day for a broken hip.

Slowly building up my self-confidence, I wrote once more to Edward with the news that I was now free. Kind as he was, he suggested we meet for a picnic on Wednesday, 19th June, my next day off.

The day arrived. I sat cautiously up in bed—and finally grasped the enormity of what I'd done. Dressing at snail's pace, I searched for an escape from the inevitable. For one brief moment I actually wished I was back in the incarcerated safety of St Francis. How could I have been so crazy? How had I written to a complete stranger, a man who lived a life light years distant from my own? A Cape Horner who was being fêted for his daring, who had been a guest on Desert Island Discs? What in the world had made me do it? What in the world would he find in common with me, already marked down as one of life's failures? While he had struggled to stay afloat in a massive storm near Cape Horn, I'd been lying with my head under a pillow, struggling to cling onto what was left of my sanity.

Distantly the doorbell rang. My stomach scrunched. I grabbed my picnic, slipped the keys into my pocket and reluctantly descended the four flights of stairs to the front door, my heart pounding fit to break a rib. There I paused. Closed doors still held a terror for me but, after all my previous bravado, I could hardly leave the poor chap outside on the pavement. I opened the door.

The man standing before me was better looking than the newspaper photograph had suggested. Wiry and about 5ft 10ins tall, he had a handsome nose, thick brown hair and a neatly trimmed moustache and beard, the latter with a distinctive white streak down the centre. Even as a small child I had found men with beards attractive. This one was wearing jeans and a blue-and-white striped matelot top. I took an instant dislike to the top, then forgot it entirely for the man smiled at me and his bright blue eyes, half laughing, twinkled in sympathy. I'm sure he'd guessed just how scared I felt.

He pointed to a blue Land Rover parked down the road. "How would you like to drive up onto the Downs? We can picnic there; find a sheltered spot and look out over the Channel."

I clambered into the passenger seat and gazed around. I'd never been inside anything as exotic as a 4 x 4 Land Rover. For some reason this one even had two small, individual motors to drive two independent windscreen wipers. Edward started the engine, and we set off with the vehicle making the most almighty racket, as if all its bolts might come flying off at any moment.

Parking the car in a layby, we took a footpath into a field, chose a sheltered corner and sat down on the grass. Way above us on the hill, a herd of young heifers placidly munched grass. Feeling awkward, I busied myself with peeling a hardboiled egg while I tried to think of something to say. I'd long since lost what little I had of the art of polite conversation.

Taking a deep breath, I finally asked, "What are you planning to do next?"

"Well, I'm here only because my father was killed in a road accident. I should be back in New Zealand with my boat. But then my mother became ill and has now died too."

I searched his face for emotion. "That's terrible. I'm so sorry."

"Yes, it came as a shock. But at least I got to see her before she died. Now my sister and I have to tidy things up and sell the house. As soon as that's done, I'll be returning to my boat."

I said nothing.

"But you know, the flight over was unbelievably tedious. That's why I bought the Land Rover. I'm planning to drive back overland. At least as far as Singapore. Bit too much water after that." And he gave me a quizzical smile.

I turned my head and gazed out to sea, contemplating his new adventure. Sitting beside him on the grass he didn't seem nearly as intimidating as I'd feared. Could he perhaps need a co-driver? I'd just decided to risk asking him when he went on.

"My girlfriend, Judy, will probably come with me. Depends on her mother. She's sick." I sat there, silent. So he had a girlfriend! Why hadn't I thought of that? To me, aged 22, 53 seemed far too ancient to have a girlfriend. Thank heavens I'd kept my mouth shut.

He continued. "I'm also legally still married. But my wife and I separated ten years ago. I've just come back from delivering furniture to her in Spain. She lives there with my step-daughter. Our daughter is here in England. She's about your age."

I was still trying to absorb this second bit of news when all hell broke loose. With whoops of glee, a bunch of stick-wielding youngsters had charged the heifers. The heifers, taking fright, were in turn charging straight down the hill towards us. I watched in alarm, thoughts careering through my head as I envisioned pounding hooves flattening us into the ground. What to do? What sort of impression would I make on this sailor-man if I took to my heels and fled, freaked out by a bunch of diminutive cows? Surely not the robust companion he needed for an overland adventure. Happily, at that moment, Edward, too, decided that retreat was the better part of valour, so we grabbed our things and scrambled unceremoniously through the barbed wire fence. Once safely on the other side we laughed together at our fright. We had survived our first joint escapade.

Regaining the Land Rover, Edward, no doubt confused by his recent trip to Spain and maybe still a little unnerved by the heifers, drove off at speed but on the wrong side of the road, provoking in me yet another adrenaline rush of fear. The guy seemed hell-bent on jump-starting my zombie spirit! Later, up in my attic, or Cave as Edward quickly christened it, I made him a cup of tea, and we agreed to meet again.

A few weeks later, Edward wrote to tell me that Judy's mother had taken a turn for the worse. Judy had decided she had to stay in England. Their plans together were over. Damned if I did, damned if I didn't and always braver on paper than face to face, I wrote suggesting I take Judy's place as co-driver.

Edward replied saying,

Dear Clare,

Many thanks for your letter. When I saw the postmark, I was pretty certain what would be inside. The offer had to come from your side. I was not going to say anything, but I felt as our views and attitude to life were so similar, it would be a pity if we just parted again, and so hoped you would offer to come. I would be glad to have you along, so let's join forces.

Later he wrote again,

"I think it's time I met your parents."

He collected me from the Cave and, on the 26th June, we drove together the twenty miles to High Beech. It was not a beautiful house, the outside walls were a cream, speckled, pebble dash, while the inside was bitterly cold in winter. Nonetheless it was the nearest thing my family had to a permanent home, and I loved it. Its eight bedrooms had come in handy when my father was sent off to war in Korea and my uncle, aunt and their two sons moved in with us. The splendid playroom, replete with threadbare carpet, had a coal fire where we could roast chestnuts or marshmallows or use a long-handled brass toasting fork to make toast for tea.

But for us children and our friends, the true glory of High Beech was its wild, four-acre garden. The 'wood', the 'moss lawns', the 'bamboo walk' and lily-padded small pond gave endless opportunities for games of hide and seek, cowboys and Indians or cops and robbers with the old, fenced-in hen house serving as a jail. The orchard filled our bellies with windfalls and blackberries, the vegetable garden provided us with secretly pilfered, deliciously sweet, raw peas, while I have already described the waterlogged grass tennis court. There were dozens of trees to climb, and in spring yellow daffodils carpeted the ground beneath my favourite spreading oak.

My parents took an immediate liking to my new friend. My father had spent his childhood messing about in boats around the Channel Island of Alderney and later in Weymouth harbour, so he understood a little of Edward's infatuation. At least more than he understood what had happened to turn his passionate, extrovert daughter into a mute psychiatric case. But then I had never told him about Hampstead Heath. Indeed I had never told anyone except Cathy—and Cathy was now dead.

That afternoon, Edward offered to entertain us with his latest slide show. As he slowly circumnavigated the globe, local yacht clubs often asked him to give a talk, and now we were going to have our own private viewing. Sitting in the darkened playroom, we were spellbound as we caught a glimpse of a way of life none of us had ever even guessed at! Tales of accidentally eating poisoned mushrooms anchored in the River Plate and storms in the Roaring Forties. Near death as he battled alone for four days and nights during a Cape Horn gale with his fifty-five-year-old yacht, *Sea*

Wanderer, severely leaking, in the end pumping out every twenty minutes to survive. On a matter of principle, Edward refused to carry a ship-to-shore radio or a lifeboat. He said, "No one ever asked me to go to sea, so I have no right to ask anyone else to risk their life rescuing me."

Next came Cape Horn bearing north with the Pacific Ocean on the left of the photo and the Atlantic on the right! Then a slide of *Sea Wanderer*, her little chimney smoking as she lay buried under a thick blanket of snow during a winter in Tierra del Fuego. Tropical pictures of Tahiti and the Tuamotus; anchored inside Minerva Reef, marked only by a wreck in the middle of the Pacific Ocean. A final shot showed *Sea Wanderer* moored in Auckland Harbour.

The playroom filled with silence as we each absorbed what we had just seen and heard. I wondered how I could ever live up to the expectations of such a fearless human being.

Brought up with two older brothers, I had always been a tomboy, racing them to climb the highest trees, defending myself in sibling fights. I think my long-suffering parents hoped against hope that this mad adventure with a man obviously able to cope with any crisis, a man they felt instinctively they could trust, might be just the thing to sort me out. They gave their blessing to our expedition and begged Edward to take good care of me. Older than my mother, did they see him as a surrogate parent? I saw him as a co-adventurer.

* * *

Soon we were meeting to hammer out our plans. Camping in the Land Rover, we would drive from England to Singapore and then, all being well, would continue by air to New Zealand for Edward to be reunited with *Sea Wanderer*. We would pack the minimum of clobber and take turns to drive—once Edward had taught me how to double declutch the Land Rover, something I'd never even heard of before.

Luckily, in my previous life, driving had been one of my great loves. As a 17-year-old, I had enthusiastically embraced it, starting lessons the first day of the summer holidays and passing my test six weeks later. I also loved Formula 1 racing and had been at Brands Hatch when Stirling Moss had his near fatal crash.

Now, of course, all sorts of advice was pouring in from friends, much of it contradictory:

"Take extra gloves, it will drop below freezing at night."

"How will you bear all that heat? Take lots of sunscreen lotion."

"You do know how to recognise a rabid dog don't you?"

"Must cover up before dusk. Mosquitos you know. Malaria."

I was still doing nights down in Hove and kept busy during the day with doctors' visits for tetanus jabs and vaccinations and having my teeth checked at the dentist.

Meanwhile, I was learning more about Edward's previous life. Soon after World War II, in fact just around the time I was born, Edward had given up his nine-to-five job as a naval architect and had chosen instead to harken to the siren's call, to sail the seven seas, to live simply and to wander the globe freely. He had earned his living in a multiplicity of ways: chartering *Sea Wanderer* to tourists in the Caribbean, doing up old boats and selling them at a profit, yacht surveying. He had run Moroccan cigarettes to Gibraltar and taken North Africa tourists out on deep sea fishing expeditions. As a qualified engineer, he had been maintenance manager for a West Indies hotel. He had also written three books and umpteen magazine and newspaper articles.

Before we could set out, Edward and his sister, Mary, also had to sort out their parents' property. Almost at the same time, Edward's spinster Aunt Ethel, died. She had owned a farm which had unexpectedly turned into prime real estate as it lay very close to where Britain's second busiest airport, London Gatwick, had recently been built. In leaving part of her money to Edward, he found himself, aged 53, with enough to live on, provided he continued to live frugally.

But that didn't help me to pay my way. At first Edward suggested that, in exchange for him covering our expenses of food and fuel, he would dictate, and I would type out, his next book. Regretfully I had to point out that I could neither type at dictation speed nor spell, so that idea withered on the vine. (It was to be another 48 years before, aged 102,

Edward published his final book, *Solo Around Cape Horn and Beyond.*) In the end we agreed that I'd be cook and caterer for the expedition—Edward hated doing both—and then, at the last moment, a friend negotiated with a Dutch magazine for me to write a series of articles about the adventure; my first writing commission, no less.

We decided to leave in July, which meant that, with little more than a month to go, I could procrastinate no longer. I was going to have to hand in my notice. I couldn't care less about my landlord nor my part-time night job with the Garage Man. It was the admirable Matron Lewis who worried me. I'd promised, only four months before, that, working part-time, I would stay a minimum of half a year. She was not happy with me but did see that this was an opportunity I couldn't miss. Nonetheless, I felt deeply guilty. A promise is a promise. Indeed, even now, I continue to feel bad about letting her down.

Meanwhile, we still had a lot to do and my experience of working nights helped. Indeed, after years of pain, I had learnt to manage on very little sleep and, to this day, I routinely wake at 2 a.m. and work until 4 or 5 a.m. before dropping off again. We agreed to meet one noon at the Iranian Embassy in London, there to apply for visas before going in search of maps.

The whole project almost foundered there and then. I arrived at the embassy around 11.45 a.m., went inside and sat down to wait. And wait. Meanwhile Edward, arriving after me, had parked the Land Rover in the street outside having spent the previous night camped by the Thames working on an article and sleeping in the van. Now he stayed in the car, sure he would spot me as I entered the embassy. He had yet to learn of my fondness for arriving everywhere early.

I didn't look out. And he didn't look in. After one hour I decided he had, very sensibly, ditched me. I got up and walked unhappily back into the street—and instantly spotted the high roof of the Land Rover with Edward positively fuming inside! Not the most auspicious start to a grand adventure. But a lesson well learnt for the future. From then on, whenever we agreed to meet anywhere, we never deviated one iota from the designated spot.

Inside the embassy we filled in our visa forms, handed over our passports and then headed for the London branch of Bartholomew's, the Scottish mapmakers founded by John Bartholomew in 1826. What a glorious place in which to conceive outlandish dreams! Here Edward bought detailed Ordinance Survey maps for every part of our journey: France, Italy, Yugoslavia, Bulgaria, Turkey, Iran, Afghanistan, Pakistan, India and finally Malaysia and Singapore. Just holding those maps in my hands turned wispy pipedreams into imminent reality.

At last, everything was ready. The long-wheel-based Land Rover had been sent away for conversion into a 'dormobile'. It returned with a red and white striped raising roof and two narrow upper bunks, one of which was for me and the other for storage. Below, the back seats folded down to form a bed for Edward.

With my previous, deeply traumatic experience of abduction and rape in the back of a van, I probably should have been afraid. But I wasn't. Over our weeks of planning, I had developed a total trust in Edward. Immersed together in the excitement and practicalities of our joint venture, he had also shown an almost missionary intent to rebuild my self-confidence and help me to recover from two years of institutional psychiatry. He himself had no time for psychiatrists, or 'trick cyclists' as he called them. As to a possible sexual relationship, at the outset I saw Edward as far too old for anything like that; not only was he some two and a half times my age but, for heaven's sakes, he was older than my mother!

Sleeping bags and pillows made up our bedding. One tin wardrobe was all we had to store our clothes. We also sneaked in such 'necessary' equipment as a stout rope for towing an occasional Maharaja's Rolls Royce out of a muddy river. And, in case the grateful Maharaja didn't materialise, we had another string to our purse. We packed my clarinet, which I was rather painfully learning to play, and Edward's castanets with which he was fairly proficient. We had grand visions of playing for our supper when we became destitute, although my clarinet playing would have to improve considerably if we were to attract coins rather than rotten eggs.

Two gas rings and a sink served for our galley with a cupboard underneath for stores. The quantity of stores I bought still makes me smile. We had bacon and marmalade and bread and butter and eggs and fruit and vegetables and jam. Anyone would think we were heading straight for Outer Mongolia rather than France, 25 miles across the English Channel. Perhaps I was a tad over-excited by the notion of our Great Expedition.

I did make one further, vital purchase. I went to my GP and asked for a prescription for a six-month supply of DF118. I was going to need those to survive the pain in my arm, which continued for a total of eighteen years.[xxxix]

Finally, we carried my few possessions down the stairs from the Cave into the Land Rover and handed back the key to the landlord. Edward drove us once more to High Beech where we dumped all unnecessary clutter in my bedroom.

My mother had invited my dear friend, Sue, and her equally dear parents, Beryl and Charles Pick, to come over for tea on our final day and to see us off. After giving the visitors a guided tour of our intrepid vehicle and giving both my parents warm, lingering hugs, it was time to leave.

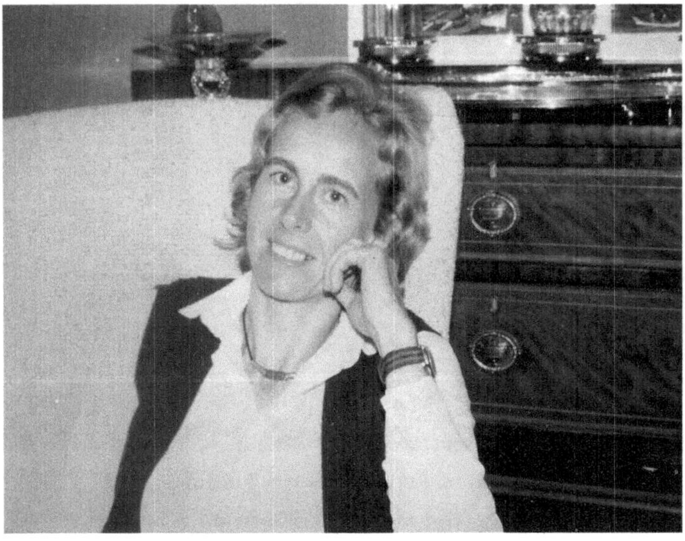

Clare in her early 20s, at her parents home.

PART TWO

TO THE DEEP BLUE SEA

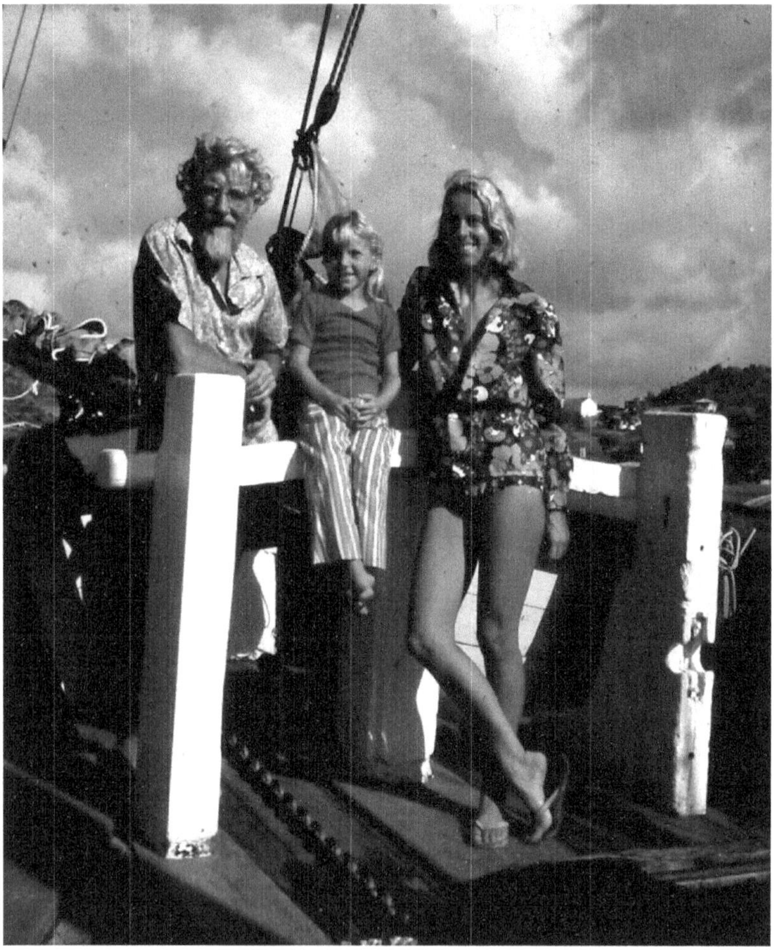

Edward, Katy and Clare on Johanne.

20

Two Drifters Off To See the World

27TH JULY, 1968. Five and a half weeks since we first met, we were almost the last to squeeze onto the night ferry from Dover to Calais. As Edward locked up the van, the ship's rear doors clanged shut behind us.

I flinch. That noise. Doors slamming shut. Metal bolts. Panic. Help! I want to get off! I won't cope, I know I won't! I'm still half-zombied. I'm not ready for this. Damn it! I'm a fantasy adventurer, a daydreamer. But that's reality out there, clanging those doors behind us. There's no pillow now for me to hide under. Worst of all, what if I fail this man beside me who, for some incomprehensible reason, believes in me enough to allow me to share in his adventure?

Did Edward sense my fear? Who knows, but he led me up to the stern railing so we could have a last glimpse of the receding White Cliffs of Dover. They looked somehow irretrievable. Then, under an overcast sky, we turned and walked to the front of the ship, towards the future, and watched the waves foaming and tumbling in their haste to escape the clean cut of the ferry's bow.

1968 and, as we drove onto French soil, signs of the previous two months of student riots were still visible in the many slogans splashed on the walls. As rain bucketed down, we followed notices to a campsite. Roof up and curtains pulled against the outside world, my spirits revived. I grinned broadly. I'd never really camped before. I'd wanted adventure and now it had begun.

There followed the first challenge—supper. When I wrote to Edward that I couldn't cook, I meant it. That night he gave me my first lesson on how to produce a passable meal on two gas rings.

Time for bed and Edward, ever a gentleman and despite the rain, said he'd just go for a walk. I pulled the curtains, had a quick wash and was tucked into my bunk under the roof by the time he returned.

The following morning, France's near-empty B roads proved ideally suited for surmounting the next hurdle in my new life as an Overlander: learning how to drive the 4x4 Land Rover, a very different kettle of fish to driving a Mini. For a start there was that double declutching to master.

Patiently Edward demonstrated.

"First you have to let the clutch *in* to shift from gear into neutral. Like this. Then quickly let the clutch *out*, and immediately back *in* again, see that? But did you hear? At the same time, I gave a quick blip on the accelerator pedal to shift into the new gear. Finally, you let the clutch *out* once more and accelerate away."

"Simple really!" I quipped.

"Now you try."

I did. I tried. But success was a long time coming. Edward would happily have driven us all the way from Calais to Singapore but he had set himself a much tougher task: to restore my independent self-assurance which lay smothered beneath two years of institutional confinement.

The terrain grew hilly, and the Land Rover's gears grumbled and growled ever deeper as they shifted downwards. We decided to name her Rumble-Tummy.

Two days later, *en route* for Genoa on Italy's Mediterranean coast, we stopped in a small town to hunt for food and fuel. Dropping me off to shop, Edward went in search of diesel fuel. I found a small grocer's and stepped up to the door. Then hesitated. I was afraid.

I didn't speak the lingo. I couldn't read the signs. But we had to eat. I had to go in. If only Edward were with me! I wasn't ready to do this on my own. Not yet.

The shop was quite full. Customers stared at me, a stranger, as I lined up at the counter. My turn came. I pointed at a baguette. The shopkeeper smiled and placed it in my basket. Milk? I couldn't see any milk. How could I say I needed milk? Stressed out, I saw no alternative. I lifted my hand as if holding, and then drinking, from a glass and, yes, I mooed like a cow. No one jeered. The women laughed—soft, warm laughter—with me, not at me. Fears unfounded, I'd survived. Basket now filled with groceries and paid for, I displayed my one word of Italian, "Grazie", and left to stand outside in the sun to wait for Edward.

That night Edward pulled out one of his favourite books, Daphne du Maurier's *Frenchman's Creek*. "Would you like me to read to you?"

"What a lovely idea!"

Curled up on top of my sleeping bag, I listened, deeply contented, as he played out the tale of love between a French pirate and Lady Dona St. Columb, after whom Edward had named his own daughter, 18 months my senior.

Television-free, over the coming months reading aloud to each other became one of our favourite pastimes. In between I was also working my way through Thomas A. Harris' best seller on Transactional Analysis, *I'm OK—You're OK*. A book that had brought help to some 15 million readers around the world as they struggled with mental illness. In it, Harris proposes that there are four attitudes to life, one of which every human being takes at any given stage in his or her existence: I'm Not OK, You're OK

I'm Not OK, You're Not OK

I'm OK, You're Not OK and, finally,

I'm OK, You're OK.

This incredible book was to have a transforming effect on my future, and I'm deeply indebted to its author. Because of Harris, I first came to realise I was firmly stuck in Position One: I'm Not OK, You're OK. How long had I been trapped there? Since being raped? Probably. But also, the attitude had been strongly reinforced by two years of psychiatric treatment when, it seemed to me, every insinuation was that I was Not OK. After all, that was why I'd been referred to them in the first place.

Except, that is, for the wonderful Dr Pirrie, the doctor who put an arm around my shoulders in the Villa and said, "You know Clare, you're OK." Maybe he'd just read Harris too? And Sister Will, whose parting gift to me that first time I left the York Clinic was to tell me that I was strong. That I could make it outside. And finally there was a moment when

Dr Christie wrote to me after I'd been transferred from one psychiatric clinic to another, saying, "I would like to wish you all the very best on your painful voyage of self-discovery and would only comment that I have always thought there was a lot you would find of value under the gilding." Maybe I should have taken that, too, as a message of hope. Instead I simply didn't believe him.

During that trip of exploration and adventure, I slowly absorbed Harris' words. Slowly grew towards being a person I could live with, I could accept. Meanwhile Edward, happily residing in the final category, was doing his very best to persuade me that I could, and should, join him there.

As we set out the next morning, Edward turned on the car radio. Up till then Cliff Richard's hit song *Congratulations* had endlessly filled the Land Rover's rattling cab. But now a new song grabbed the airwaves: *Moon River* from the film, *Breakfast at Tiffany's.*

"...You dream maker, you heartbreaker..." I turned my head and gazed at the man beside me. Was it possible? Was this *my* heartbreaker? *"Wherever you're going, I'm going your way!"* That was certainly me. *"Two drifters off to see the world, there's such a lot of world to see."* And that's us!

I leant over to get his attention. "Do you hear that, Edward? This is 'our' song!" and I touched his hand lightly. Edward's hands were beautiful: sensual, sinewy, dusted with fine fair hairs. And in that moment, a bolt of sexual awakening flashed through me. Something totally unforeseen was happening. I was tumbling in love with an eccentric, wise, rebellious, kind, enigmatic, funny, occasionally short-fused, devil-may-care adventurer more than 31 years my senior.

Entering the city of Genoa, we went in search of the hotel where an elderly Italian yachtsman had reserved us a room and a space in their locked parking area—pretty imperative as the van was carrying nearly all our needs for the next 9,000 miles to Singapore. He had also invited Edward—'famous yachtsman'—to dine with him the following evening at Italy's oldest and most prestigious yacht club, the Yacht Club Italiano, founded in 1879. No way was I going to join them there.

Parking the dormobile, we entered the hotel lobby and crossed to the desk. The receptionist looked up and asked matter-of-factly, "Double or two singles?"

I looked at Edward, a shy question in my eyes. He returned my look, his own eyes smiling, one eyebrow raised in query, a slight shrug of the shoulders. It was up to me to decide.

I paused. Fear flushed my cheeks while the words "Hampstead Heath" whispered in the echo chambers of my mind, a horror about which Edward knew nothing. But must that one incident blight my existence for ever? Was it not time to move on, to embrace a new life and satisfy a nascent hunger? Could I find the courage to say yes?

I turned to the woman. Took a deep breath. Stared coolly into her eyes and said, "A double please."

That night, after the luxury of a hot bath, we tumbled together on the hotel's wide white bed in a delicious release of pent-up desires. As dawn broke, I mused over the fact that, in English, we say lovers "sleep together". As far as I could make out there was very little sleep involved.

It was then, as I lay, curled up with my head on Edward's bare chest, his sheltering arm around me, that for the second time in my life, I put into hesitant words what I could remember of Hampstead Heath, an experience so terrifying and humiliating—and so utterly different to this.

From Italy we penetrated the Iron Curtain and arrived in Yugoslavia. An immigration official came out of his booth and asked if there were just the two of us. I nodded. Then I whispered to Edward, "He's probably looking for my chaperone."

"But surely I'm the one that needs the chaperone!" Edward joked, eyes twinkling.

From then on, all the anti-communist propaganda dissolved before us. What wonderful, laughing, friendly people. The first night we camped on a fishing village's tiny jetty. And within minutes there was a tap on the window. A beautiful young teenager presented us with a dish of steaming fresh-caught fish cooked over some bits of wood right beside us on the dock. An impeccable ambassadress for her country.

In stark contrast, Bulgaria measured up perfectly to Western propaganda which, till then, I had discounted as extreme. Here were glum faces, drab clothes. At the border we were each handed a grey, lined card to be filled in, stamped and signed each night by the guard of one of the country's official tourist camps. And it was here that I discovered that Edward didn't believe in rubber stamps or officials and had absolutely no intention of searching for a government campsite.

"That's it! I've had enough! All this official campsite stuff is perfectly ridiculous!"

And he pulled off the road to park for the night hidden beneath the branches of some apple trees.

I hate raised voices, and I detest fights, but Edward's determination not to stop in an approved campsite was, in my opinion, just asking for trouble, especially under a communist regime that we knew nothing about. And it was a sign of how far I had journeyed since first meeting Edward, that I dared to remonstrate at all.

"But who knows what sort of trouble we'll be in when we leave the country? Maybe they'll throw us in jail! We must find a proper campsite." My voice turned squeaky with alarm as I warily watched his expression. What would he do? Shout? What a wimp I'd become since being in hospital, intimidated by the consequences of daring to rebel. I lost the argument. We stayed beneath the fruit trees. The balance of power between us remained frustratingly one-sided.

Next morning we set out eastward, ever eastward, now heading towards the Black Sea. The date was the 21st August 1968, quite a momentous date as it turned out. As we aimed for the capital, Sofia, in search of the British Embassy and our waiting mail, I spotted a group of low buildings set amongst acres of agricultural land. A Communist co-operative farm no less. Maybe I should send a picture back to my young nieces? So Edward stopped the car. We climbed out and took photos.

We were preparing to leave when a gang of hostile farm workers poured out through the imposing entrance gate and surrounded us. We were trapped. And scared. Without running them over we couldn't move. Finally, from down the road came the sound of soldiers marching towards us, guns and all. My fears redoubled. With belligerent hand signs, the soldiers ordered Edward and his camera out of the van.

I watched, helpless, as they marched him back the way they had come, leaving me alone in Rumble-Tummy with the crowd staring at me like a zoo exhibit. Fearful of attack, I quickly locked each door, no central locking back then. What now? What could I do to rescue him? What if he didn't come back? I felt adrenaline spinning through my brain. But then a wave of anger pushed out my fear. How dare they kidnap Edward? Defiant and fuming, I climbed into the back of the van. I'd thought up a particularly nasty revenge.

I unearthed my clarinet. I didn't play it well. Indeed, I hardly played it at all. But I rammed the different parts together and, flicking through my teach-yourself-the-clarinet book, I chose two tunes which I proceeded to play *fortissimo*. First *The Battle Hymn of the Republic* then *God Save the Queen*. That would teach them! And it did. They fled. Whether it was my subject matter or the sheer awfulness of my playing that did the trick I did not know, nor care, but finally I was left alone to wait—and wait—for Edward to reappear. What if he didn't? This, for me, was a constant fear lurking at the back of my mind. That somehow, in the middle of nowhere, where I could not speak a word of the language, we would become separated. I would have no means of communication. No way of finding him and virtually no money.

Eventually Edward returned, this time with only one soldier as escort. "I've got news for you," he said as he clambered back into the driver's seat. "Last night the Soviet Union invaded Czechoslovakia! Our little Bulgarian brothers suspected us of spying."

Somewhat chastened by this experience, Edward finally decided we'd better search for an official campsite—and found a really rather nice one, right on the beach beside the Black Sea.

The nightmare of Edward's arrest, followed by the huge relief of his release, had brought us yet closer together, converting our Great Adventure into something more like a Great Honeymoon. We lazed together on the sand, swam together in the warm sea, walked hand-in-hand along the beach—and slept together on the fiendishly uncomfortable 'double bed' created by sliding the Land Rover's two folded-down back seats together.

Happiness! I couldn't remember ever feeling such happiness in all my life. It welled up, unbidden inside me, pressing against my diaphragm till I could barely breathe. This surely couldn't be reality, but an illusion encircled by a rainbow-tinted bubble of delight. One day soon the bubble would burst, and we would step out into the world and into Life. But, hopefully, not until our present journey was over.

Two days later we headed for the border. For nine days I had worried about what would happen when we handed over our grey cards. Edward was totally oblivious. In the event our treatment was almost an anti-climax. The immigration officer skimmed down the pages where, luckily, all four camp guard signatures came one after another with no flagrant gaps in between. He added our cards to his pile and waved us through. I admitted, grudgingly—and secretly—that one could say Edward had been right.

But this journey was teaching me something else. Something very important. To live in the moment, not agonise all the time over a future that might never come. That so often, in the end, my fears were unfounded. And if something did go wrong, well maybe I could cope. After all, when needed, I'd seen off angry farmers single-handedly. Each day, our experiences were making me stronger.

Crossing from Bulgaria into Turkey, I found the contrast between the two countries quite baffling. Just over the border, a group of small Turkish children smiled and waved enthusiastically. I could scarcely believe it as I smiled and waved back. Then their mothers joined in! Could it be that we were actually welcome here? Why so different? How could a few hundred meters of No Man's Land so radically change human temperaments? Was it because Turkey had spent millennia as a crossroads, a trade route; that the Turks were used to welcoming strangers? Or was it that Bulgaria's repressive regime had stifled the natural generosity of its people? Or maybe it was simply a difference in trust. Maybe, like me, the Bulgarians had grown afraid to trust.

I fell in love with Istanbul on sight, a city afire with energy. Anarchic traffic poured in all directions whilst pedestrians stepped fearlessly out into the road with complete disregard for the dolmuşes, a sort of communal taxi, that hooted peevishly as they swerved past.

To the east of the city, the roads rapidly deteriorated till it was hard to decide which was worse: swerving around giant potholes or juddering over the dirt trail's iron-hard corrugations. We pushed valiantly on at a coccyx-crunching 26mph—only to be confronted by a notice forbidding us to exceed 55mph. They must be joking! At that speed our brains would have scrambled inside our skulls and Rumble-Tummy would have snapped a halfshaft—a sadly unreliable part of Land Rovers at the time.

The roadways, though very wide, only had a single track down the middle used by traffic. Vehicles from both directions vied with each other to take possession of that central lane and a battle of nerves ensued to see who would blink first and swerve onto the rough. I blinked quite often.

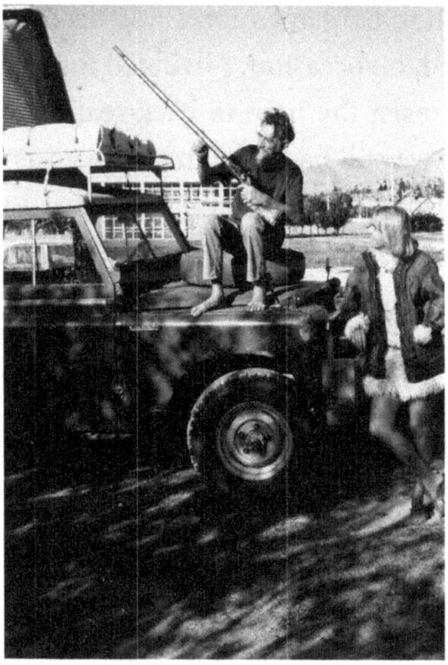

Edward with a flintlock, Clare in an Afghan coat.

21

Journey's End and a New Life Begins

As we travelled east, the heat inside the Land Rover became stifling and the tempers of its two occupants somewhat frayed. I have since decided that a relationship that can survive months shut up in a boiling hot metal box, nine feet by five, can probably survive anything. Poor Edward! His ideal travelling companion, the one who barely opened her mouth, was changing. His determination that I should once more grow confident was bearing fruit. As we drove towards the rising sun, so my robust self re-emerged from under the grey clouds which, three years before, had fallen from the sky and crushed me.

For him, I became once more a stranger, someone he had never met till now. He, along with the excitement of the journey and Thomas Harris' book, was healing my broken psyche—and in return he was perhaps getting more than he'd bargained for. I was becoming opinionated and argumentative—and, on occasion, I irritated the hell out of him.

If only he could resist the urge to back-seat drive! Bad enough on a shopping spree but we still had 4,000 miles to go as the crow flies—and we weren't crows. I had to try to remember that I wasn't the only one bringing baggage into this relationship. Edward, too, had scars left over from a stormy marriage that led him to opt for ten years of solitude. It couldn't be easy after that decade of freedom, in which he did exactly what he pleased, to then share his life, his space—and a very small space at that—with someone else. At least the clatter of Rumble-Tummy bumping, diesel-powered, over the rough roads, made conversation difficult and prolonged arguments rare.

Suddenly, the road deteriorated alarmingly. Somewhere people must have endured an earthquake, but we had no way of knowing where.

For we had, for several weeks now, lived in a media blackout, unable to understand either local radio or newspapers. For all we knew, France had become a dictatorship of the student masses, and the US had been invaded by the Viet Cong.

Many bridges were down, obliging us to ford rivers, a nerve-wracking business with no marker posts to indicate the depth ahead and with water rising above the hub caps. At one place we had to wait for bulldozers to clear a landslide. At another we stopped while a man hammered a hefty new plank onto a primitive bridge. We had quickly learnt that it was imperative to take those rural bridges at precisely the correct angle, or one could miss the two stout planks provided for our wheels. Further on we found half the mountain track had tumbled into the valley far below.

Mid-afternoon I pulled off the road and, using the 4x4, bumped over the stony ground to stop beside a large rock lapped on one side by a swiftly flowing river. An ideal setting in which to sample the joys of nature's washing machine. I'd grown to love scrubbing clothes in rivers and by now had become quite expert. For a start always place the garments to be washed *upstream* of you. That way, if the river goes into tumble mode and a wavelet snatches away your knickers, you are in a position to field them before they disappear downstream forever.

It was dark and the moon was rising as I finished draping the clothes on prickly bushes to dry. A cool night breeze whipped the hair from my face as I stripped off and bathed in the shallow water.

Is it something primitive inside me, maybe inside all of us, that fills me with such exultation; to be here surrounded by the night silence, alone beneath the stars and the moon so far from home? Happiness swells within me, takes over my whole being until it's bursting to escape into the universe, leaving but a wraith behind.

For some time Rumble-Tummy had been climbing and we stopped as the sun hung just above the mountains on Turkey's 6,250-foot high Kara Bayir Pass. The view was spectacular. In front of us was a thousand-foot drop and across the cloud-strewn valley we could see Kose Mountain rising 11,736 feet into the deep blue sky.

I went to sit cross-legged on the edge of the abyss, to drink in the mystic beauty of the place. I was elated, *aux anges!* Completely at peace, gloriously alone. Just me and nature perched on the edge of the void.

And then suddenly, rising from that self-same void, it returned. It filled my head, shushed in my ears, that terrifying sense of compulsion, the feeling that I *must* kill myself, that it was my *duty* to launch myself into the chasm, to wipe the evil that was me from the face of the earth. I thought I'd got it vanquished. I thought the journey had put an end to that driven madness of guilt and shame, but no, it was I who had to do that. I who had to put an end.

I stood up and for a long, long time gazed down at the dark shadow of land far below. I swayed on the edge, wavered, conflicted, torn.

And then I turned and walked slowly back to the van and Edward. It was over. With no going back, I had chosen Life.

It was in Iran that we finally learnt about the earthquake, the evidence of which we had come across way back in Turkey. It had been massive, with some 16,000 fatalities, its epicentre close to the holy city of Mashhad. Could we perhaps help?

Being a holy city, I took extra care to dress modestly: long sleeves, long skirt and a headscarf to cover my hair. We found the Red Crescent offices but were informed, regretfully, that our lack of Farsi meant that we could be of little use. That settled, we went in search of a new inner tube for one of the tyres. Edward parked on the edge of a roundabout and set out on foot, leaving me behind to keep guard.

He was barely out of sight when a gang of youths, maybe university students, swarmed around Rumble-Tummy. They pulled open the passenger door, and, as I tried to grab it shut, one hit me over the head. With no central locking, I scrabbled to lock the doors. Then they started to rock the Land Rover, building up momentum in an effort to turn her over. I was petrified. On the far side of the roundabout I could see a policeman. And he could see me. But he made no effort to help. Neither did pedestrians passing by. Were they, too, frightened of the mob?

At last my frozen brain jerked into action. Hadn't Edward left the keys in the ignition? Unlike Iranian women, I could drive. I slid swiftly behind the wheel and switched on the ignition. To my great satisfaction, the youths jumped back in disbelief. Then, keeping in neutral, my teeth gritted in wrath, I stamped the accelerator pedal full force against the floor. Rumble-Tummy roared in full throated fury. The men cringed even further back. What victory! I'd done it. And done it all on my own. Me against a gang of youths. Wow! I felt so strong and empowered and self-confident.

Then, putting the dormobile into gear, I set off round the roundabout glaring ferociously at the useless policeman. But where to go? Edward had to be able to find me. In the end I snuck down a side road, hoping I was close enough for Edward to spot me as he searched. And there I waited until he eventually returned.

* * *

We were nearing the Afghan border, and I was driving along a perfectly good, hard topped road, when Edward, gazing at the map, noticed a tiny, dotted line. A Caravan trail no less. How romantic! So much more fun than a boring old tarmacked road! And so off we charged in a cloud of dust along a single sandy track into the desert. But then, an hour or two later, the single sandy track divided into seven sandy tracks—and not a signpost in sight. We were completely lost. But thank goodness for my sailor-man, famous for having a solution for every occasion. Edward rummaged once again through his little safe-box, took out a compass—and we made it to the Afghan border by compass course.

Dusk had fallen and the border was about to close as we finally left Iran bound for the kingdom of Afghanistan; the most rugged and, for me, the most eagerly anticipated country of our Grand Adventure. A few miles into No Man's Land we pulled over for the night. By now we had spent eight and a half weeks on the road and travelled some 6,000 miles.

Afghanistan! It didn't disappoint. The most enjoyed of all our destinations. Wonderful wild, proud nomads. Incredible Hindu Kush mountains and of course the legendary Buddhas of Bamiyan. Sculpted 1,400 years before, one of them stood as high as a 17-storey building.

That night, all around us, the landscape lay flat and flinty-silent while, above, remote stars pierced the dark canopy of heaven. Yet sleep wouldn't come. As I lay beside Edward, anxious thoughts chased across the night sky of my mind.

For it was there, in Afghanistan, that I knew I was definitely pregnant. Edward had run out of condoms in Bulgaria. Searching our Bulgarian pocket dictionary we found no entry for 'condom'. And frankly, they are not something that exactly lends themselves to either sign language or the odd sketch. We decided instead to try the rhythm method, and the rhythm method had failed.

I had a life-changing decision to make. And yes, Edward made it very clear it was my decision. He would back me whatever I chose.

In 1968 only 17% of children were born outside wedlock, and those children were labelled 'illegitimate' and 'bastard'. Unmarried mothers were still a subject of shame to their families. As I listened to the silence of the Afghan night, I lay torn between hope and fear.

Hope because I loved children; my first job had been as a mother's help. All the other thoughts teaming through my brain revolved around fears, haunting fears that luckily most women never have. *What if I suffer post-natal depression and, once more, they lock me up? Depression makes a sorry home for any child. And what happens when Edward sets sail once more on his single-handed circumnavigation? I had no right to wreck his life-long dream and beg him not to go. Still, it would leave us all alone in some strange land, our child and me.*

Finally, what of my parents? Hadn't I caused them enough disgrace without this? First mad and now pregnant? Was it perhaps my duty to have an abortion? Was that the kindest thing to do? For both the child and them?

As part of my nurse's training, I'd worked a stint in theatre. Soon after I started the secondment, I was attached to a young gynaecological surgeon. He had spent the whole morning doing D & Cs which involved scraping the tissue lining from women's wombs. My job was to fetch and carry while the theatre sister handed him the instruments. But then, soon after I started, as one anaesthetised patient was wheeled out and another was about to be wheeled in, Sister turned abruptly to me and said, "Nurse, I would like you to scrub-up for the next operation." And she left the theatre on some errand. I felt honoured that I, so new to theatre, had been briefly entrusted with her job.

As the young surgeon and I diligently soaped and scrubbed our hands and forearms under the hot running water, he said vehemently, "God, this is one operation I loathe!"

My eyes opened wide. In that case why do it? Why spend all morning doing a conveyor belt of D & Cs on women suffering from polyps or fibroids or heavy periods?

Neither of them saw fit to warn me that I had been elected chief assistant at an illegal abortion.

When the young doctor scoured out the tiny foetus with his sharp, long-handled curette, it was already perfectly formed; only, in removing it from the womb, he had accidentally torn off one minute arm. He then had to fish around in the dark cave of the woman's uterus to recover it. He laid the arm reverently on the green surgical cloth covering the patient: amputated, complete with its five tiny, translucent, perfectly formed, pink fingers. He carefully inspected the body for any further mutilation then placed both foetus and arm gently in a kidney dish and gave it to me to dispose of. I can see that defenceless little arm to this day.

In the end, I decided to listen to my heart. I wanted this child of mine, and I would keep it. Along with writing that first letter to Edward, it was the best decision of my life.

So, I knew about abortions and yet I didn't believe that they were invariably wrong. Aged 22, I had already come across too many people permanently damaged as the result of being either an unwanted child or a desperately overburdened mother.

One woman I met lived with her husband and their two small children in a one-roomed flat. Pregnant with a third child and at her wits' end, she went to her GP to beg for an abortion. He refused. Shortly afterwards, she threw herself out of their third-floor window. She and her baby were killed. Her other children left motherless, her husband a widower.

By now we were both getting pretty road weary. We still had the great subcontinent to cross and then the drive down the Malaysian peninsula to Singapore. But New Zealand, *Sea Wanderer* and Edward's continued solo circumnavigation called.

We covered the remaining ground as fast as we could. Managed to book on a ship sailing from Madras to Penang in Malaysia followed by a very pleasant drive down that beautiful peninsula full of shading trees and neat, clean *kampongs* of wooden houses raised on stilts.

In Singapore we booked Rumble-Tummy onto a cargo ship and, on the 3rd December 1968, we finally flew the last 10 hours to Auckland.

There we quickly fell into a routine, basically working seven days a week to get *Sea Wanderer* ready for her next great voyage: carrying Edward, alone, some 7,000 miles northwest around Australia to Singapore. He, along with John Ryan, an unconventional and talented carpenter, treated *Sea Wanderer*'s 58-year-old hull with a new deck and several new planks. Meanwhile I became expert at scraping old paint down to the bare wood, sanding it, treating it with preservative before repainting the boat inside and out. I found it incredibly satisfying seeing the tired old yacht transformed and looking quite new and young again. Which was just as well as I was eventually to do the same sort of maintenance on our various vintage boats for another 35 years.

It must have been in March 1969 that Edward and I went into Auckland to see the film *Oliver*. Seven months pregnant, when the film's interval arrived, I got up to head for the lavatory. At that moment I felt a tap on my shoulder. I turned round, and there, right behind me, stood Dr Pirrie; the psychiatrist from The Villa who had been the first to tell me I was okay, who had taken me to the talk on contraception because I might "need it one day".

How perspicacious was that? And what a mind-blowing coincidence that, half a world away from the UK, he should be sitting directly behind me in a cinema! He indicated with a sideways jerk of the head that we should meet outside. Poor man, what could he have thought seeing me there, heavily pregnant and accompanied by a wild-bearded man double my age? His kind eyes questioned me, full of anxious concern.

"Don't worry, Dr Pirrie. Really!" I smiled up at him. "I'm the happiest I've ever been in my whole life. That man in there's amazing. We've just driven for four months from the UK to Singapore in a Land Rover. The adventure of a lifetime. And we're madly in love and this is our child," I said caressing my bump with pride. "Thanks to Edward and the journey and Thomas Harris book, *I'm OK. You're OK,* I've finally accepted that I'm OK too, neither devil nor saint. Just normal." And I beamed at him with delight, before turning and going swiftly back to sit next to my beloved dream maker.

And I was okay. So much potential had been strangled that night on Hampstead Heath. Strangled by fear and then suffocated by silence. Never again would I bury terror and shame alive. I had learned a vital lesson. Deep trauma must be shared, if only with one other person. And hope. Never lose sight of Hope. Through all that nightmare my parents had clung steadfastly to hope, to their belief in my capacity for health and happiness. And now that capacity had been unlocked and filled with joy, as I stood on the threshold of a new life. I had finally learnt to accept myself as I was and that, I believe, is the foundation of all mental health.

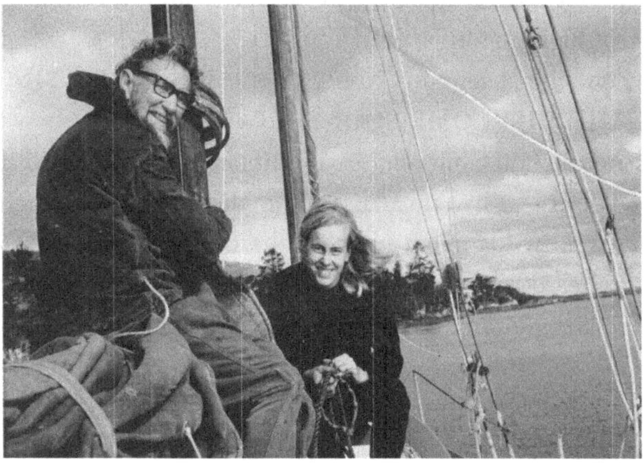

Edward and Clare on Sea Wanderer.

How Life Went On[XL]

AUCKLAND TO EAST TIMOR

OUR DAUGHTER KATHERINE Helen Allcard, a healthy bonny 8lb baby, was born on 27th May 1969. A natural birth, it took the two of us just six hours from start to finish. I was told the next one would be born while I was still standing at the kitchen sink. Was it due perhaps to all that vigorous scraping and painting and bending and standing of the past four months? Then, some five months later, Edward set off on the second half of his solo circumnavigation. Strong and independent now, Katherine and I were to join him in Portuguese Timor, Singapore, Seychelles, South Africa and finally Antigua where in 1973 he completed what some people have called the slowest ever solo circumnavigation.

Once Edward had left baby Katy and I in Auckland, we had no means of communication until he reached his next stopover. He was bound for Singapore and our plan was simple. On receiving a telegram saying he'd arrived, I would buy a one-way ticket, turn what was left in our New Zealand bank account into travellers' cheques, collect our few belongings not already aboard *Sea Wanderer* and, together with Katy, take a direct flight to Singapore.

But when the telegram came, it read: DELETE SINGAPORE SUBSTITUTE DILI COME SOONEST. Well, I'd try my best to follow Edward's instructions, but *Dili*? Living in a temporary rented flat in the Auckland suburbs, I had no atlas and no idea where the wretched place was. Panic was swiftly followed by Bright idea! Go to a travel agent! But she'd never heard of Dili either. It would be another thirty years before the verb 'to Google' would become my knee jerk reaction to almost any query. However, after several phone calls, the travel agent managed to track the place down. It was the small main town in a tiny Portuguese colony occupying the eastern half of the island of Timor, just across the Timor Sea, north of Darwin, Australia.

So, in 1969, aged 23, along with babe-in-arms Katy, we had first to fly to Melbourne, spend the night in a B&B, then taxi to the airport for a flight to Darwin right at the northern tip of Australia. Once again into a B&B to wait for the weekly flight to Dili in a six-seater, twin-prop Cessna. By now, money was becoming a major concern. We had enough money in our local bank account for the single flight to Singapore, but would it cover flying from Auckland to Melbourne, then Melbourne to Darwin and finally on to Dili?

Well, it did—just. Arriving in Darwin with virtually no money to spare, I searched out the very cheapest B&B. Our room was minute. A cracked basin served for washing and a small window looked out onto a vacant lot. Located just 12° south of the equator, the heat was horrendous. But let's look on the bright side. The menu for the breakfast part of the deal was a page long. And, if so inclined, you could order the lot at no extra cost! The lack of any refrigeration made me choose carefully: cereals, scrambled eggs, and toast and marmalade for breakfast, with salad and other, slightly less perishable things set aside for lunch and, finally, lots of bread and cheese and an apple for supper. I was still breastfeeding six-month-old Katy, so I had to make sure I ate a healthy diet.

Finally, the time came to catch the weekly flight to Dili. The Cessna pilot couldn't have been kinder, helping to carry Kate's in-flight necessities on board, stowing everything away and checking that I was firmly buckled up and my little one safe. The flight was quite bumpy, but actually that was a good thing as it seemed to lull Katy to sleep. At the time she was going through a rather tedious stage of screaming her head off—without tears—whenever her will was frustrated, such as when I put her in her crib for the night. Happily she decided that flying was OK.

The flight distance from Darwin to Dili was around 700 miles, by which time I was totally exhausted. And anxious. I hadn't heard from Edward since the original telegram. Would he be there to greet us? Had he even received my telegram with our ETA?

Peering out of the window as we landed on a rutted field, I spotted a hut. And there, standing in front of it, was my beloved Edward, the most compassionate yet fearless man I have ever met, and blessed with a contagious wit to boot which kept us both smiling. Wiry, with twinkling, sky blue eyes, gold-rimmed glasses and a brown beard with a distinctive white streak down its centre, my darling man was right there, his arms waiting to welcome us.

It turned out that Edward had anchored off Dili because the seasonal fair wind for Singapore had petered out. Over the years of globetrotting in Edward's wake, or at his side, I discovered that this happened more often than not, especially as *Sea Wanderer* had only a diminutive engine and just a little diesel for Emergency Use Only. So basically it had to be 'Up sails!' or 'Down anchor!'

But these wind changes also brought exceptional rewards. Over some thirty years roaming the oceans in two quite different wooden sailboats, we spent more than six months waiting for the wind to change in New Zealand, Portuguese East Timor, Singapore, Malaysia, Thailand, Sri Lanka, Chagos archipelago (illegally), Seychelles, Kenya, South Africa—where we paused for a moment to get married—Antigua, Grenada, Spain, France and England and amongst all those there was only one country neither of us planned to return to. That was Perim, a Yemeni island at the southern entrance to the Red Sea, where we were briefly held captive.

Dili, on the other hand, was fabulous. It had sandy lanes for roads and mainly bicycles for transport. Located close to the famous Spice Islands, it is mountainous with the lower slopes and the plateau leading to the sea, covered with a rich variety of tropical trees: coconut, oleander, rubber, sandalwood, tamarind, toddy and jackfruit to name a few. In Timor, a deeply Catholic country, Katy caused a major sensation. Many had never seen a blonde baby before, except on religious cards, where, for some unknown reason, baby Jesus was usually depicted with blond hair. The poor child had to put up with frequent passersby touching her head for good luck!

We lay, anchored off Dili, for six months, waiting for the wind to change and so, bit by bit, we made local friends. Back in Portugal it was the time of the right-wing dictator, António de Oliveira Salazar, and we quickly discovered that this remote colony was where he exiled his left-wing political opponents. Which also accounted for the inordinate number of soldiers roaming the sandy streets. On top of which it elucidated the weird restrictions placed on any visiting yachtsman, or wandering hippy for that matter, wanting to visit us on board. What did they think we were doing there? Secretly planning to whisk some deserving exile across the seas to freedom?

Meanwhile, as we met other people so often at the Miramar Hotel, I also got to know the manageress. A tall, elegant woman, originally from Goa off the west coast of India, we struck up a friendship and she became like a doting grandmother to Kate. Which meant that the young waiters were allowed to play with her too. They loved to pick up the blonde baby and carry her around.

Ashore, a short walk from the hotel, was a crèche run by Portuguese nuns. Feeling it would be good for Katy to see other babies and for me to do some volunteer work, I went along to offer my services. Even today East Timor is one of the most impoverished countries in the world and of all the places I've visited, it was only here at the crèche, that I saw such pathetic, Oxfam-thin children. There was one main cause behind this: the colonial government's levying of taxes. Taxes most Timorese could not afford. At the crèche there was one child so thin that, at age five, she weighed less than Katy aged nine months.

Finally the wind changed fair. It was time for Edward to leave. Standing on the beach, Kate in my arms, we waved goodbye as he set sail once more for Singapore. Katy and I moved ashore into one of the Miramar's little, shady, guest bungalows. The following day at the crèche, one of the nuns said rather archly to another in Portuguese, "I hear Joseph has left." To which I quickly chirped up, "Yes, but Mary and Baby Jesus are still here!" Poor loves, how they tittered, not sure whether to be embarrassed or amused.

NAIROBI TO THE SEYCHELLES

The next divergence from an expected itinerary came when Katy and I were living in Kenya's capital, Nairobi, three *months* after Edward's expected arrival in the country's largest, Indian Ocean port of Mombasa. Three months of complete silence, as he sailed alone some 3,200 nautical miles from Singapore and across the Indian Ocean to Africa. Complete silence, which gave me plenty of time to imagine every possible, horrific scenario: had the boat sunk? Had he been attacked by pirates? Or killer whales? Had he died of a heart attack? We might never even know, maybe he had just vanished from the face of the earth?

Meanwhile, two-year-old Katy and I had been staying with my sister-in-law Helen, my brother John and their five children. This was in the expectation that Edward would sail into Mombasa a couple of weeks later and that, while waiting, we would have fun getting to know each other again and Katy could play with Georgina, her senior by three months and the youngest of her five cousins. However, remembering Benjamin Franklin's famous adage "Guests, like fish, begin to smell after three days", the longer we waited the more sensitive and anxious I became.

And then, on 12th December 1972, a truly extraordinary thing happened. It was around lunchtime and Helen suddenly turned to me saying, "You're going to hear from Edward today!" I mean, she could have said that, with the same deep conviction, any time over the past two months. We worked out later that she had actually said it as Edward was sending off a telegram saying: "DELETE MOMBASA SUBSTITUTE SEYCHELLES COME SOONEST HAVE FOUND LOVE NEST"

Sadly, "Come Soonest" turned out to be impossible. He had chosen the era when the Ugandan dictator, Idi Amin, was expelling all the country's long term, Asian residents back to the Subcontinent. Every steamship heading east from Mombasa, towards the Seychelles and Bombay was packed with refugees. And at that time the Seychelles had no airport.

Which is why Kate and I had to go the 'long way round': fly to the UK, fly to Bombay and then catch one of the now empty refugee boats back to the Seychelles' main island of Mahé. I can feel to this day the powerful wave of joy that rolled over me as I stood on the steamship's upper side deck, Katy in my arms, peered down to the water—and spotted Edward almost alongside the ship in our rowing dinghy.

A couple of days later, we upped anchor on *Sea Wanderer* and set out on the 25-mile crossing from Mahé, heading for La Digue, the third largest island in the archipelago, and home to the promised 'Love Nest'.

Back then there were no cars on the island. Come to that there was no running water or central electricity either. But what it lacked in utilities La Digue made up for with its amazing, unspoilt beauty. Walking along the sandy track which served as the only road, it probably took us 20 minutes to the plateau where the Love Nest was located, with nothing but palm trees between it and the sea.

As we walked up to the house my heart welled up with delight. It was gorgeous! A wooden hut built on stilts, in the vain hope of fending off termites. The Love Nest had a deep, sloping, palm thatched roof with a balcony along the length of the wall looking towards the beach. Walking round to the side, I climbed up a flight of three wooden steps to open the door. Not as easy as I had expected, the rusted, iron hinges screeched in pain as I wrenched them open—and stopped dead. Clearly Edward hadn't visited for some time for all over the floor were four-inch-high pyramids of wooden dust, dust created as termites ate the hut's main beams. I turned to Edward, exclaiming, in mock indignation, "This is no Love Nest, it's an Ants Nest!" And so, it remained for the next ten years or more.

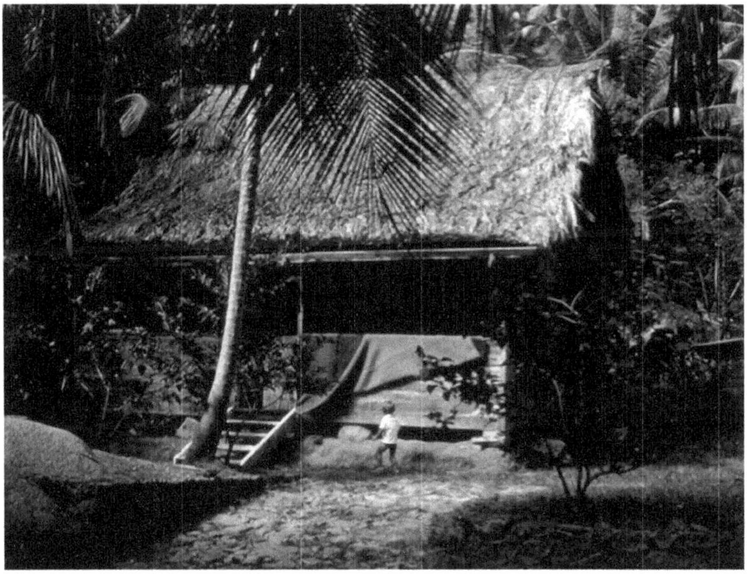

The Ants Nest.

DURBAN

At the time of Kate's birth, children born outside wedlock were still quite rare in the UK, though becoming more and more accepted. My worry, at the time, was that the trend might one day reverse, leaving Katy unfairly stigmatised. It was for that reason that we decided to get married. The question was, when?

Divorce laws in the UK had become much more accommodating and since Edward and his first wife had already been separated for ten years there was little problem in getting one. By the time Edward had sailed the 2,000 odd nautical miles across the Indian Ocean from the Seychelles to Durban, South Africa, *Sea Wanderer* needed to be hauled out of the water for considerable repairs so, leaving young Katy with my doting parents, I flew out to Durban to be with my beloved Edward.

And it was there that we decided to tie the knot, choosing the registry office of a small town in the Drakensberg Mountains called Mooi River. Why? Simply because the name sounded so like our favourite song, 'Moon River'.

Edward, famous amongst yachtsmen for always having useful gadgets to hand, realised we were going to need a wedding ring. No problem, he had just the thing. Disappearing below he came back with a metal wire tray of family trinkets, medals etc, amongst which were two gold wedding rings: one his mother's and the other his grandmother's. I no longer remember which one we chose. Our honeymoon was brief but glorious, in the stunning scenery of the Drakensberg Mountains. When Edward eventually died in 2017, aged 102, we had, disproving all the nay sayers about our age gap, been together for 49 years and a day.

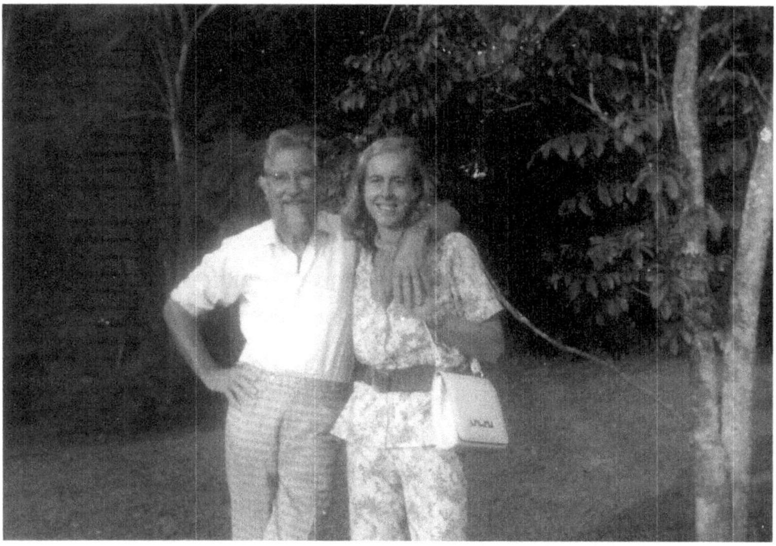

Edward and Clare Allcard, married at Mooi River.

ANTIGUA

Katy was four, the circumnavigation was complete, *Sea Wanderer* was being prepared for sale, and we were living ashore in English Harbour, Antigua, when Edward first set eyes on the 'dream ship' that would become our family home. She had just been hauled out of the water for repairs.

Edward already had a long-term dream—to build a replica of Columbus's sailboat, *La Niña*. He'd even cut most of the wood for her, now seasoning on our little coconut plantation in the Seychelles. With her, we planned to take part in period films like 'Mutiny on the Bounty'. Until that is, everything changed.

With Edward and Katy, I clambered aboard the Dream Ship (at that point called *Edith M*) and watched as my husband paced out the boat's length on deck, 69ft and her beam 20 ft, sized up her draft, or depth below the waterline: 7 foot and the result was, quite frankly, amazing. She had almost exactly the same dimensions as those Edward's friend and naval architect, Colin Mudie, had drawn up for him from an illustration of *La Niña*! With just one major difference—the present boat was already built.

Major repairs were clearly in order. For a start, over the past six months, the 69ft wooden ship had lain sunk in English Harbour, slowly dying from neglect. The sinking was due to the fact that the young owner and his crew, who had bought her in Denmark and sailed her across the Atlantic to the West Indies had, on arrival, been caught smuggling drugs. The men were arrested, and she was abandoned with a police writ on her mast: a sort of handcuffs for boats found complicit in crime. And of course, over the months, the protective, underwater, antifouling paint lost its potency and delighted wood worms crowded round to snack eagerly on her naked planks. It was due to them that she sank.

A classic Baltic trading ketch, our dream boat boasted two pinewood masts, the taller, main mast, some 70ft high. Then there was her magnificent 18ft bowsprit raked out in front of her bow, which was more slender than on most Baltic ketches, and painted the traditional black. An elegant pirate ship no less!

Built in Faarborg, Denmark in 1929, we discovered she had had quite a remarkable history over the years, including a number of name changes, thought by sailors to bring bad luck. Due to the First World War, there were any number of trading ketches to be found laid up along the coasts of Denmark waiting for peace and commerce to return. But, for merchant sea captain Jensen, none of them was quite what he wanted. He decided to build a new vessel to his own specifications. With very few others at the time interested in building brand new cargo boats, he had the pick of the very finest woods. After a lengthy search, he managed to find one beautiful, solid oak tree to serve as her keel. Later, as we replaced much of her ancient, worm-eaten 3-inch-thick planking, we discovered magnificent oak frames beneath, a good man's fist wide, they rose like giant whale's ribs, they were so close together. And, as if that was not enough, on the inside of the frames there was another layer of oak planking sealing the interior and intended to protect the cargo hold from any leaks. Those Danes sure knew how to build sturdy boats.

However, there was one snag. Edward had fallen in love with her just after she had been bought by a most remarkable West Indian, Mrs Matthews. This extraordinary woman, maybe in her sixties, living ashore in a wooden house with a corrugated iron roof, had quickly seen the boat's potential, bought her as a wreck and renamed her *Edith M* after herself. She had purchased the ketch for her sons to start an inter-island cargo business. With help from the harbour master, she arranged for the boat to be hauled out of the water and slid up onto Antigua Boatyard's slipway—where Edward had spotted her.

After only a few months, the cargo business had collapsed. As *Edith M*'s leaks had not been fixed, sea water inexorably rose inside the hold ruining her various cargos of cement and sugar and household furniture. When Edward stepped onto the scene, Mrs Matthews was in luck.

Approaching his new beloved from the stern, I could instantly see her attraction. She had the finest transom, tucked up and heart-shaped. Less attractive were her wood worms and they were just the start of this Noah's Ark collection of livestock, none of which, by the way, had come in two by two. There were rats everywhere and revolting swarms of big, brown, flying cockroaches with long, twitching antennae. Indeed, on second thoughts, maybe *Edith M* wasn't so alluring after all. But the more we delved into her history, the more fascinated we became. So much so that we decided, once we had made her seaworthy, we would sail her across the Atlantic to her Danish home port of Faaborg, a mere 3,000 nautical miles away. At this point we still didn't even know her original name. We idly speculated on her hull, unusually slim for a cargo boat. Was she originally a smuggling ship? Smuggling gold? Or spies? Not that she was exactly fast. But all these things are comparative.

FAABORG

Many months later we motored in between the high sea walls protecting Faaborg Harbour on Funen Island. I still remember the internal terror of that moment. As our 18ft bowsprit poked into the harbour, I realised the place was chock-a-block; no room for another dinghy, let alone 68ft and 99 tons of Baltic trader. I was standing in my place, up forward, ready to drop the anchor if and when commanded. A few minutes later Edward shouted, "Let her go!" I did, but frankly with heart in mouth! I had huge faith in Edward's seamanship but now, with yachts and ships all along the harbour walls, some worth hundreds of thousands if not millions of pounds and with their anxious captains watching our every move, I let the anchor go. As the heavy anchor chain rattled out, Edward waited a moment to let the anchor reach the bottom and then put the engine hard astern, digging the anchor into the mud and stopping the boat in her tracks. She then swung slowly round to face into the wind. And as she swung, we passed so close to some of the moored yachts that I could have shaken their captain's hand. But we didn't touch a single one. Some of the yacht crews (I suspect in relief) actually gave Edward a round of applause.

After supper and a good night's rest, we went ashore in search of our treasured foundling's history. The harbour master directed us towards a little upstairs bookshop, near the harbour entrance. The shop was full of nautical sailing books. Hundreds of them. The owner, a man in his late 60s, greeted us in English. Edward explained that we were in search of information about our Baltic trader. He immediately pointed out of the window in the direction of *Edith M.* "Ah, do you mean the *Maria* out there?"

Wow! Just like that. It turned out he had a book in Danish all about the trading boats that had been based in Faaborg. What's more, he knew the widow of the first owner and their son and also the fabled captain, Kartoffle Jensen, or Potato Jones (the Kartoffle being in honour of his cargo.) No spies, no gold, but perishable potatoes and other vegetables picked up from Denmark's many islands and carried to the capital as swiftly as possible. She was called the *Maria* as the owner called all his boats *Maria*. But after passing her on to his brother, it was the brother who first named her Johanna. I think it must have been the English owner, when trying to register her in the UK, found that the name Johanna was already taken and so he named her *Johanne Regina*, or Queen Johanne, a beautiful name for such a much-loved Dream Ship...

THE CHAGOS ISLANDS AND SRI LANKA

Johanne Regina was our home but slowly, over the next several years, we made our way gently back towards that small holding in the Seychelles where we believed we would finally settle. We were in no hurry, but by the time we finally reached the Seychelles there had been a communist coup. A 6pm curfew had been imposed, and new laws let the government to seize any form of public transport without compensation, and that included *Johanne*. Bitterly disillusioned, we felt forced to leave. In May 1980 we sold our beloved Ant's Nest and headed north towards Sri Lanka. Katy, aged 11, was due to start school in England in September. There was just time for one more grand adventure.

1000 miles away in the middle of the Indian Ocean, lay the islands of Chagos, leased as a naval base to the United States. The Americans in turn put this out of bounds to the rest of the world. Chagos became the cruising fraternity's forbidden fruit. With two extra crew, Sylvie and Anne, *Johanne* set out in what we expected to be a ten-day voyage. Battered by gale after gale, it took twenty. But once arrived all the effort and anxiety proved worth it. For six weeks we lived a Robinson Crusoe existence, roaming the empty beaches, collecting coconuts, catching fish, diving the magnificent coral reefs and of course repairing all *Johanne*'s recent gale damage.

Each day US fighter jets buzzed us, flying low over *Johanne*'s masts and shattering the silence of paradise. Then one day, a naval vessel appeared outside the lagoon. We were ordered to leave.

Sailing north again, we made landfall in Sri Lanka. Once moored, Edward and I went ashore to complete the formalities and search for mail. An immigration officer at the port gates asked. "Have you daughter of doctor on boat?"

Yes, I said. Anne's father was a doctor.

"She have letter. Father dead."

I looked at him in horror. Anne adored her father, a gorgeous man and dear friend of ours. We hurried to collect the mail. Then came an even worse shock. The dead man wasn't a doctor at all. He wasn't Anne's father. He was my father. They had buried him a month ago, but we had no ship-to-shore radio, so we didn't know.

Kate and I flew to England the next day. I silently weeping the whole way. My father, aged 70, had been rude good health when I last saw him. Then an embolism from a hip replacement had killed him in seconds. We stayed a month with my mother while I tried to comfort her, and then together she and I installed Kate in boarding school. On her very first evening. Kate met another new girl who had also been homeschooled, was also wearing flip flops and who had grown up on a Malaysian oil palm plantation. Those two 'Third Culture Kids' became fast friends. I flew back to *Johanne* feeling I had lost not one, but two members of my family.

SINGAPORE TO ANDORRA

We spent the next four years cruising the coastal waters of Singapore, Malaysia and Thailand, while searching for the best hardwoods, boatyards and shipwrights. On three separate occasions, we had to outwit pirates. But apart from the pirates, the tropical sun was beginning to take its toll. After years of living in the open without using sunscreen, Edward developed precancerous skin lesions across his shoulder. I, meanwhile, was getting heartily sick of being groped in streets by local young men. It was time to return to Europe. But where?

For the second time in my life, fate intervened in the form of a newspaper. On this occasion, it was wrapped around a baguette. As usual, once home I straightened it out and read it. It bore an advertisement from CISA, an estate agency based in a place called Andorra, a place I had never heard of. Edward, on the other hand, had. He even seemed mildly interested.

Since leaving the Seychelles *Johanne* had been our only home. Maybe it was time we invested the money from the Ants Nest in another small house? The next day I went to the hotel where CISA was exhibiting photos of Andorran properties. In the course of chatting, they showed me a picture of a little place standing all alone in an alpine meadow with a pine forest stretching up behind it up to white mountain peaks. Even more important, they told me that Andorra required no visas.

I raced back to Edward with the news. And two weeks later, I flew to Europe with a list of criteria from my reclusive husband: must not be able to see another house, must not be able to hear a dog bark, must not be passed by heavy traffic. Almost all houses in Andorra are in building clusters and most clusters appeared to have at least one barking dog, but eventually we came to a little orchard surrounded by communal land that could not be built on. No dogs, no traffic. And, provided you looked in the right direction, no houses. A few months later, we signed a contract with CISA to build us a house.

Leaving the sea and our travelling life took time, but we finally moved to live in Andorra in 1987. Once there, one of our first actions was to ask immigration about becoming passive residents. The female immigration officer could not have been kinder. She was truly concerned that after so many years living with wide horizons, we would feel hemmed in by the mountains. Edward replied poetically. "Oh no. It's all nature. Mountains are just waves standing still."

For the first time since leaving the UK, I could become deeply embedded in a local community. I helped found a choir which today boats fifteen nationalities. I started a writers' group. Became a hospital volunteer. I felt I belonged. In 2016, together with friends, I published *Andorra Revealed.*

During the first decade of our new life away from the sea, I completed *The Intricate Art of Living Afloat* and also wrote *A Gypsy Life.* Then I set myself the challenge of writing this book. I had become enraged by the judge's infamous verdict in the 1986 Ealing Vicarage Rape case. Jill Saward and her boyfriend had been visiting her father in his vicarage. There was a ring at the door. Jill went to answer it—and was held at knife point as three burglars forced their way in. They proceeded to tie up and then bludgeon both her father and boyfriend with a cricket bat, fracturing their skulls and rendering them unconscious. Next, two of the three dragged 21-year-old Miss Saward upstairs and gang raped her.

My outrage came when the presiding Old Bailey judge, Mr Justice Leonard, sentenced the burglar who did not rape her to fourteen years in jail and the two younger robbers who did, to five and three years for rape and five for burglary. The judge then had the gall to turn to Miss Saward and tell her that "her trauma had not been so great".

In fairness I should mention that, until then, Mr Justice Leonard had had a good record for thoughtful sentencing and, forever haunted by the public reaction to this one judgement, he made a public apology to the victim on his retirement. Nevertheless, then and there I made a note to myself that I would write a book describing the consequences of my own traumatic abduction and rape.

I had not kept a diary, but the memories were still very live. My brother David had died in 1992 and his widow returned a box of our correspondence. I have always been a hoarder of family letters, and I still had the letter sectioning me. I never did tell my parents about being raped. Indeed, until I decided that I had to write this book, I had only ever told Cathy and Edward. Now I wanted to explain the devastating effect that the terror and revulsion can have on a woman's life.

My closest family—Edward, Kate, Dona—supported me. I had learned so much more about PTSD and the importance of talking to people about traumatic events. The more I think about it, the more I am convinced that the PTSD came from him pretending to throttle me, and my being convinced, at that moment, that he was going to kill me. So convinced that when I saw the blanket I put two and two together, and saw it as death with my body wrapped up inside. They say that PTSD is frequently caused by coming face to face with what looks like imminent death. My mother wrote 'reminding' me that, for months afterwards, I woke every night crying out in terror. I, in fact, remember nothing about that at all.

I think now that this has all been laid to rest, yet sometimes still I feel people draw away a little when I say that I was raped. And I am still making progress on the terrible shame that I felt at being so stupid as to put myself in that situation.

* * *

When I finally started work on this book, I wrote to my mother asking her to tell me how this journey of mine had appeared from her point of view. Here is her wise and perceptive reply.

<u>FROM MY MOTHER</u>

From the beginning you were the much-wanted daughter and a child after my own heart! Enchanting to look at, full of fun, amenable to discipline and apparently by far the easiest of my children to bring up...

You seemed to take your various schools in your stride, always bubbling over with chat about them and apparently telling us everything that happened. You seemed to make a lot of good friends and be willing to take responsibility. But then the arm came and lack of sleep and bad dreams. Looking back, I don't think we should have encouraged you to do nursing (though you seemed so cut out for it) when you had that constant, nagging pain.

I didn't get really worried until you started the psychiatric nursing and you came back obviously upset and anxious. [That was right after I was abducted and raped. I never told her what happened.] *Again, looking back, I probably ought to have got on to someone and said I thought you were feeling the strain, taking your responsibilities too seriously.*

Now to try to sort out my feelings. <u>NO</u> resentment—I have never thought why should this happen to me? About you or anything else—though this seems to be quite a common reaction. Things happen in life, and it is what you make of them that matters.

Of course we wracked our brains as to what could have caused it, and what we had done wrong, but honestly I don't think I felt I was to blame. You and I had seemed to get on so well with very little of the teenage alienation, and certainly I thought this might have been part of the trouble, that you hadn't gone through the rebellion stage at the right time.

As to what I said to people, it was that you were suffering from depression, mental breakdown and one soon found that a number of others were in the same boat, either personally or with members of their family. Except for Cousin Lorn and Beryl [Sue's mother], *I don't think I told people in so many words that you had attempted suicide. I found nothing but sympathy from people, and surprise that it should have happened to you, but then I have fairly remarkable friends on the whole. The prayers of my religious friends may not have done any good to you, but they were a support to me.*

One's relationship with the psychiatrists was distinctly mixed. Knowing nothing about it one had to rely on them in the first case especially as you were at the York Clinic with a good reputation. We agreed to the ECT and then, as that didn't seem to work, to that extraordinary month of 'deep sleep' when you were only wakened for about two hours in the twenty-four to be fed.

But then they did such daft things, like letting you out and telling you to get a job at the very particular time when we had told them not to because Dad was going to be at the other side of the world, and only a short time after the 'deep sleep'. And then again in January, telling us to find you a job on a farm in mid-winter!

We thought all those places in Brighton and Hove appalling and no help to you—and the Villa not much better—but when it came to the crunch and you were attempting suicide one only had the psychiatrists to turn to.

After your last attempt, they told us that they were moving you over [to St Francis], *on Section, because it wasn't fair on the Villa nurses to find you in pools of blood or running away and possibly falling in front of a train. I remember Wheeler saying that you had got to rock bottom and could only go up from there.*

I think we always thought you would get better in time, and probably irrespective of what treatment you were given, as long as we could prevent a successful suicide. So it was when you were in digs that was the worst time. Also feeling so helpless—why couldn't I think of the right thing to say or do to get you out of it? The psychiatrists were hopeless at giving us any advice on how to treat you though, on the whole, they seemed to think it was probably better to visit than not to visit. So, although it was heart-breaking to see you so miserable I thought it was important to keep contact. But maybe, as it only increased your feeling of guilt, this wasn't a good idea?

Anyway enough! I hope that has answered your queries to some extent. I haven't ever talked to you about it because I wasn't sure how good it would be for you to go over all that blackness. But if you are doing so anyway, then it doesn't matter.

Looking Back and Then Forward

Looking back on those years—the simulated strangulation and rape, the buried terror of coming face to face with death followed by the trauma of PTSD, the later attempts at suicide, the psychiatric hospitals and then the treatments—I feel I have finally come to terms with them. They remain in my memory, a strange, desolate part of my life, but no longer in 3D. Neither are all my thoughts negative from that time, maybe because I had the luck to be born naturally positive. I was a very cheerful child, with two, much loved and loving parents. I don't ever remember hearing them angry with each other or raising their voices, though I do remember my mother sometimes being exasperated. Life cannot always have been easy for her, an army wife with three children, frequently on the move. I remember also a special moment, whilst visiting my parents in their small Georgian house on the outskirts of a Sussex village, when the front door bell rang. I went to open the door to a man from Christie's London Auction house. He walked in, paused, then said, with pleasure, "What a wonderfully happy house!"

It was partly the rape, but even more, the fear of imminent death by strangulation that tipped me into a whirling, suicidal black hole but I think the time in the York Clinic, The Lady Chichester hospital, The Villa and the White House Day Centre also brought positive changes into my life along with widening my horizons and giving me a deeper understanding of human nature,

Today, my first thanks go to my fellow inmates. Far from being shouting crazy or somehow dim, as painted in two dimensional descriptions of psychiatric patients, the great majority in fact formed one of the most intelligent group of people I have ever lived with. Privately sharing with patients who had trodden parallel paths and with a code of absolute secrecy attached to anything one shared one-to-one, finally gave me space to confront my own recent traumas, without fear of being judged and in an atmosphere of complete trust that gave me space to reconsider my own life and reactions. And, after my beloved husband Edward, it is those patients that I thank foremost for my recovery.

And yes, my psychiatrists: Dr Stead, Dr Pirrie and Dr Christie all played an important role too. Showing as they did, incredible patience while trying to persuade me to unpack my trauma instead of attempting to throw away my life.

I remember Dr Stead once asking me, "Tell me Clare, when are you going to stop running away from us and your past?"

"When there's nowhere left to run to." I replied. Indeed, it was a phrase I once considered as a title for this book.

All that said, it was in fact two men who led me finally to view myself not as some deeply evil outcast, possibly in danger of destroying the entire planet, but as an acceptable human being with the ordinary hangups found in most humans.

The first of those two men was, of course, my future husband, Edward Allcard, who set me firmly on the road to psychological health. Unlike me and my fellow patients, Edward wasn't in awe of psychiatrists or diagnoses, he accepted me as an individual with an unusual life story: no shame, no fear. Someone whose natural compassion urged him to nurture. Indeed I sometimes wondered if he saw me a bit like a human version of one of his bedraggled but beloved wooden boats, in urgent need of love and rescue?

I never actually met the second man who made an indelible impact on my life. Thomas A. Harris M.D. was the author of the bestselling book that I took with me on our overland trip to Singapore in 1968. Basically the title says it all. *I'm OK, You're OK* was first published in 1967. Through word of mouth, five years later the book made it to the New York Times Best Seller list and remained there for almost two years. It was estimated by the publisher to have sold over 15 million copies by 2004 and to have been translated into over a dozen languages. Several of those copies were bought by me to be handed on to friends, young and old, whom I met along the path of Life and whom I felt could benefit from Dr. Harris' wise insights.

And then there was Katy, or Katherine Helen Allcard to give her full name. Born to us in New Zealand in 1969, until she was 11 she travelled the world with us. Sadly suffering from motion sickness: swings, ox carts, cars, busses and, most of all, boats, she never once complained. Happily, in port she was usually just fine but we never dared take her across an ocean. Instead her deeply loving maternal grandparents would fly out to wherever we were and carry her home to England while Edward and I made our next voyage.

That is, until the anti-seasick medicine, Stugeron, entered our lives and everything changed. Though, because we still never dared take her across an ocean, her very first action after leaving school was to hitch hike from the UK to Gibraltar and find herself a job crewing on one of the yachts entering the transatlantic OSTAR race. Later she worked aboard various charter yachts in the West Indies, ending up skippering one, before deciding that what she really wanted to do was to canoe solo across Northern Canada. Once there, she first got a job taking tourists down one of the world's most spectacular rivers, the Nahanni. Then she travelled back east, bought her own canoe, put it in the water at Churchill on the Hudson Bay and paddled the Mackenzie River back to the west coast. In the process she met her future husband, Eckhard Krabel, also canoeing solo to the west.

My beloved Edward skied until he was 92, then died in 2017 aged 102. Tragically, eleven months later, our fabulous, adventurous daughter, Kate, died from genetic cancer, but not before she'd canoed alone across northern Canada. She was 48 and left a husband Eckhard and two sons, Franz and Flynn.

And as I write this, I have their two adult sons, my grandsons, on a short visit before setting out to bicycle 300km in two days across Turkmenistan. Those adventurous genes are still running strong in the family's veins.

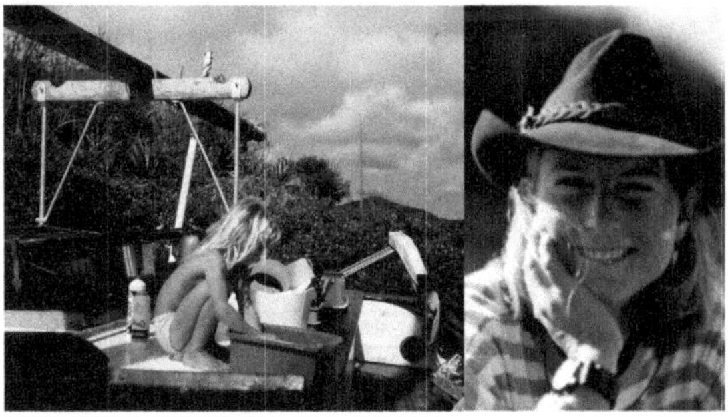

Katy: on the left, doing her chores, moored amongst the mangroves in Antigua; on the right, as an adult.

Acknowledgements

FIRST AND FOREMOST my thanks go to my dear Sis, Dona Mackereth, who not only designed the brilliant cover of this book, capturing as it does both the chaos and then the final joy of my life after I met her amazing father, Edward, but who has also encouraged and supported me during the years it has taken me to put our story down on paper. A tad older than me, I never think of Dona as my stepdaughter but as my dear, dear friend, so wise and calm and generous.

I also want to thank my publisher, Julia Jones, whose fascinating book *Stars to Steer By*, serendipitously brought us together and whose astute suggestions lead to the book you now hold in your hands.

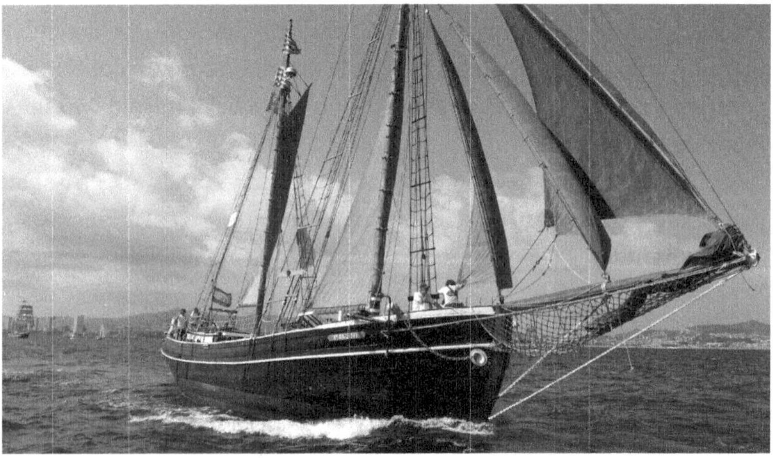

Johanne *in Badalona. [Credit: Ciutat Badalona]*

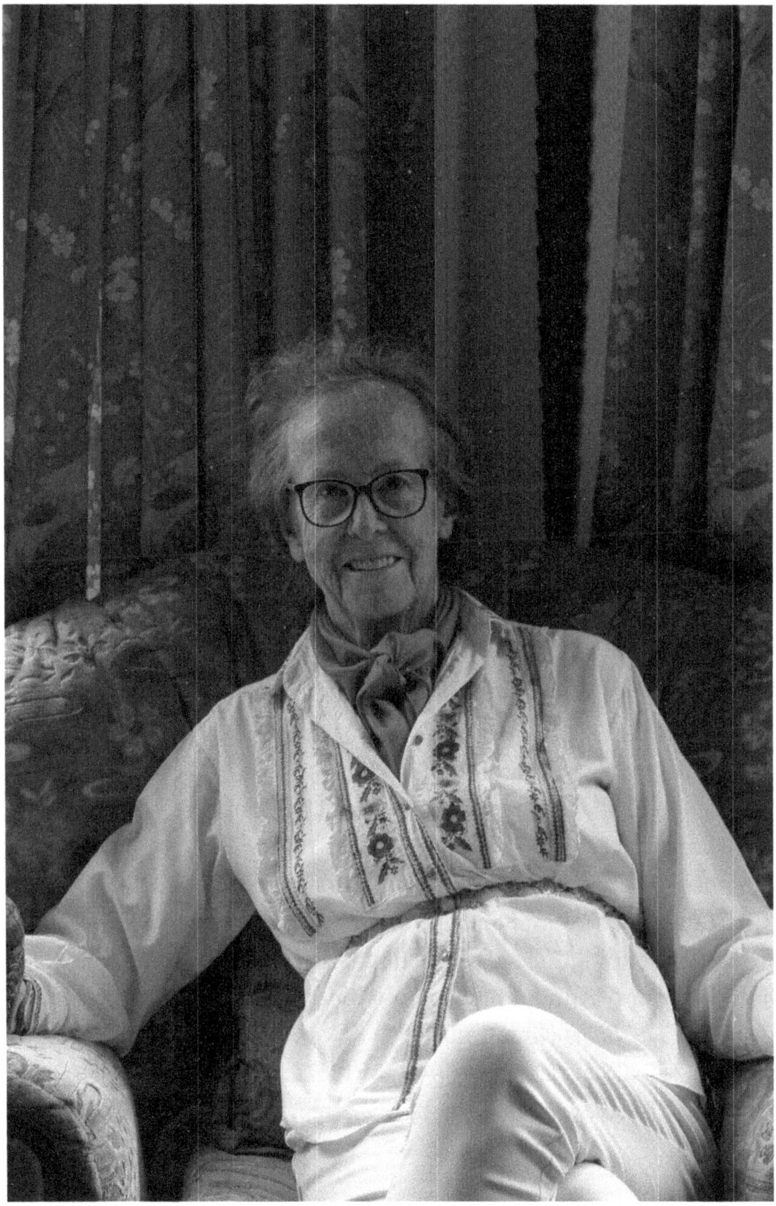

Clare today. [Credit: Flynn Krabel, Clare's grandson]

Bibliography

BOOKS BY CLARE ALLCARD

A Gypsy Life (WW Norton 1992, new ed. Imperator Publishing 2016)
The Intricate Art of Living Afloat (WW Norton 1990)
Andorra Revealed (lead author with others) (WoolyAllWood 2016)

BOOKS BY EDWARD ALLCARD

Single-Handed Passage (WW Norton 1950)
Temptress Returns (Putnam 1952
Voyage Alone (Dodd, Mead 1964)
Solo around Cape Horn and Beyond (Imperator 2016)

BOOKS CONSULTED IN PREPARATION OF THIS VOLUME:

Russell Barton *Institutional Neurosis* (John Wright 1966)
Charles Doane *The Boy Who Fell to Shore* (Latah Books 2022)
Phil Fennell *Treatment Without Consent* (Routledge 1996)
James Gardner Sweet *Bells Jangled out of Tune: A history of the Sussex Lunatic Asylum* (Brighton 1999)
Linda Gask *Out of Her Mind* (Cambridge University Press 2024)
Ed Gorman *Death of a Translator* (Arcadia Books 2017)
Thomas A Harris *I'm OK – You're OK* (first published USA 1968)
Claire Hilton and Tom Stephenson *Psychiatric Hospitals in the UK in the 1960s* (Royal College of Psychiatrists Witness Seminar 2019)
Joe Hughes *My Asylum* (Bothán Publications 2015)
Tom Lee *The Bullet* (Granta 2024)
Barbara Robb *Sans Everything* (AEGIS 1967)
Jon Stock *The Sleep Room* (The Bridge Street Press 2025)

Endnotes

i St Francis Haywards Heath, founded 1859 as Sussex County Asylum, closed 1995.

ii Email to editor 17.7.2025.

iii Quoted Tom Lee *The Bullet* (Granta 2024) from Diana Gittins *Madness in its Place: narratives from Severalls Hospital 1913–1997* (Routledge 1997).

iv Ed Gorman later discussed his compulsion to head for the sea as part of his recovery, with his psychiatrist, Dr Mills. "One of the interesting things is that anything to do with water calms the right side of the brain down. So what you were doing was seeking out water to calm your right brain." Death of a Translator (Arcadia Books 2017)

v The Woodside psychiatric unit was in Muswell Hill. It closed in 2010. Information from *The Lost Hospitals of London* https://ezitis.myzen.co.uk/stlukeswoodside.html

vi Clare now believes that she was suffering Post Traumatic Stress Disorder (PTSD). This was not accepted into the list of formal diagnoses until 1980.

vii Wikipedia https://en.wikipedia.org/wiki/Rachel_Pinney

viii Clare had been brought to the York Clinic, a tall building on several floors, part of Guy's Hospital, London. Photo and further information see https://www.researchgate.net/publication/8186411_War_and_the_Practice_of_Psychotherapy_The_UK_Experience_1939-1960 by Edgar Jones

ix Dr Fleminger obituary https://history.rcp.ac.uk/inspiring-physicians/john-jack-fleminger

x Dr Ian Christie later became a pioneer of therapeutic drug and alcohol recovery programmes https://www.phoenix-futures.org.uk/about-phoenix-futures/meet-phoenix-futures/our-history/

xi Dr Stafford-Clark wrote a brief memoir of his life and his time at the York Clinic https://www.cambridge.org/core/services/aop-cambridge-core/content/view/0D9177A9BB60EE2B513E9E3DF568022A/S0140078900017168a.pdf/div-class-title-perspective-an-hour-of-breath-div.pdf

xii Founded 1919 for treatment of shell-shock victims. From 1948 it was situated at Ham Common and pioneers the concepts of group therapy and psychosocial nursing.

xiii Dr Fleminger's first clinical lecture at Guy's was on Hypochondriasis. (source 'Psychiatry at Guys' by Dr J J Fleminger *Guy's Hospital Gazette* 1983 p296)

xiv This second operation took place at Hurstwood Park Neurological Centre, Haywards Heath, in the same grounds as The Villa and St Francis Hospital.

xv Chapter 11 of *Treatment Without Consent* by Phil Fennell identifies the mid

1960s and early 1970s as a period when voices, other than the patients' own, began to question the lawfulness of treating psychiatric patients without their consent. There was also awareness of the potential for additional 'treatment' as punishment.

xvi Article by Dr Fleminger in Guy's Hospital Gazette 1983 refers to deep narcosis as a "standard practice" at the York Clinic (p301)

xvii Sue Pick, daughter of literary agent and publisher Charles Pick. Later married Partap Sharma https://en.wikipedia.org/wiki/Partap_Sharma

xviii Fuff, Timmy and Gee were Grace, Winifred and Gladys Foster.

xix Dr Stafford-Clark (article cited above) was proud that he and his colleagues at the York Clinic "were among the pioneers of general anaesthesia and muscle relaxation for ECT".

xx Largactil was chloropromazine, hailed as a wonder drug in 1950s. An effective anti-psychotic, it avoided the need for physical restraint

xxi A letter, in which Clare's mother describes her feelings, is included at the end of this book (pp228-230). Jon Stock's book *The Sleep Room* (Bridge Street Press 2025) has examples of parents sending their daughters to Dr William Sargant at the Waterloo Clinic (attached to St Thomas's Hospital) for deep narcosis in order to persuade them to modify their behaviour or forget undesirable boyfriends. The York Clinic has issued an apology to any patients who were harmed by Dr Sargant's use of this treatment (*The Sleep Room* p256).

xxii Sometimes referred to as "the long hot summer" of 1967 it was a period of race riots in the USA but was also known as the "summer of love".

xxiii Clare's father, Brigadier WFK Thompson, served in the army for 30 years then became defence correspondent for the *Daily Telegraph*. https://en.wikipedia.org/wiki/William_Francis_Kynaston_Thompson

xxiv Dr John Sumner Stead (1918–1998) was consultant psychiatrist for the Mid Sussex hospitals https://history.rcp.ac.uk/inspiring-physicians/john-sumner-stead

xxv *Sweet Bells Jangled out of Tune: A history of the Sussex Lunatic Asylum (St Francis Hospital) Haywards Heath* James Gardner (1999) is a history of St Francis Hospital from 1850s to its closure in 1995.

xxvi Maura Hughes has her own memory of this doctor and his empathy for those in pain.

xxvii The Lady Chichester Hospital was a pioneering psychiatric facility founded in 1905 by Dr Helen Boyle for the treatment of neurosis. It was closed in 1988. More information and a comment facility can be found https://www.mybrightonandhove.org.uk/places/placecivic/lady-chichester-hospital/lady-chichester-hospital

xxviii St James's Portsmouth, Dr Christie established 'Europe's first concept-based therapeutic community' here https://austinpublishinggroup.com/drug-abuse-addiction/fulltext/ajdaa-v1-id1003.php

xxix Britain's oldest mental hospital. Then based in Bromley.

xxx Clare remained in touch with 'Hannah' for many years. Her friend eventually committed suicide.

xxxi Clare was writing in 1990s.

xxxii Lithium compounds can be used in the treatment of bi-polar disorder, particular manic episodes https://en.wikipedia.org/wiki/Lithium_(medication)

xxxiii St Francis had been suffering problems recruiting female nurses, partly due to pay and conditions, partly to the stigma of working in such institutions. From the late 1950s they attempted to solve this problem by recruiting nurses from the Commonwealth (Gardner p269). Many also came from Ireland.

xxxiv Uncle Bill was William Cobb, clinical neurophysiologist, National Hospital, Queens Square https://collection.sciencemuseumgroup.org.uk/people/ap28731 Corresponded and worked closely with EEG pioneer William Grey Walter https://en.wikipedia.org/wiki/William_Grey_Walter

xxxv James Gardner, who was a porter in St Francis in the early 1970s, quotes a newspaper interview with Dr Wheeler April 1969 'The hospital is only suitable for 700 patients but we have 900 .... There is not opportunity to give people the privacy or decent conditions that anyone would expect. The effect of conditions here must be to dehumanise patients. The conditions are an affront to human dignity.' (Gardner p275) In *My Asylum* Joe Hughes gives more detail about living and working conditions from a nurse's point of view.

xxxvi Name changed.

xxxvii In *My Asylum* Joe Hughes includes a long and reflective interview with Dr Wheeler (p169) as well as with other members of staff from this period. As a student nurse in 1967, working in The Villa and St Francis main building, when Clare was a patient there, he was earning £5 a week once board and lodging had been deducted. (p153)

xxxviii Newspaper interview with Dr Wheeler (9.4.1969) included his comment that understaffing meant that 2 or 3 time a month a member of staff was attacked on the disturbed wards. (Gardner p275)

xxxix The pain from a trapped nerve had begun when Clare was 13 and had reached her full height of 5'8". Even after the operation which finally remedied previous errors, the pain did not immediately cease, and she needed to continue taking DF118 (dihydrocodeine) for a while longer. Although this was an opioid she experienced no addiction or withdrawal problems.

xl This section was not part of Clare's original book but has been compiled from her other writing, published and unpublished.

Maritime Titles from Golden Duck

The Yachtsman Volunteers Collection:

- *The Cruise of Naromis: August in the Baltic 1939*
  GA Jones
- *Man the Ropes: The Autobiography of Augustine Courtauld—Explorer, Naval Officer, Yachtsman*
  Augustine Courtauld
- *From Pole to Pole: The Life of Quintin Riley*
  Jonathon Riley
- *Maid Matelot: Adventures of a Wren Stoker in World War Two*
  Rozelle Raynes
- *We Fought Them in Gunboats* (HMS *Beehive* edition)
  Robert Hichens
- *Scapa Ferry*
  Antony Bridges

The Lionesses of the Sea Collection:

- *When I Put Out to Sea*
  Nicolette Milnes Walker
- *My Ship is So Small*
  Ann Davison
- *The Seabird*
  Rozelle Raynes
- *From the Devil to the Deep Blue Sea*
  Clare Allcard
- *The Tuesday Boys*
  Rozelle Raynes

The Strong Winds Series by Julia Jones (with illustrations by Claudia Myatt):

1 *The Salt-Stained Book* (available as an audiobook)

2 *A Ravelled Flag*

3 *Ghosting Home*

4 *The Lion of Sole Bay*

5 *Black Waters*

6 *Pebble*

7 *Voyage North*

Books by Claudia Myatt:

- *Anglo-Saxon Inspirations: Designs to Colour and Create*
- *One Line at a Time: Why Drawing Is Good for You and How to Do It*
- *Sketchbook Sailor*
- *Antarctic Sketchbook*
- *River Deben Colouring Book*

For a full list of Golden Duck titles, including the Allingham family series and the *Please Tell Me* activity books for older people, see our website golden-duck.co.uk.

Most titles are also available as ebooks.

You may additionally be interested in *Uncommon Courage: The Yachtsman Volunteers of World War II* and *Stars to Steer By: Celebrating 20th-century Women who Went to Sea* by Julia Jones, published by Adlard Coles. Both are alternatively available as audiobooks.